ADVANCE PRAISE

"Annie Spencer's bravery to speak the truth [   ]
forward, away from both the 'suffering addict' and victim-blaming dis-
courses that surround the opioid crisis, and reminds us that there is so
much more behind the death and destruction of illicit opioid use and
accidental overdose in the United States. Weaving together personal experiences, socioeconomic analysis, and historical insight, *How to Break an
Addiction* invites us to look at this whole mess differently and reframes
addiction and chaotic substance use as a consequence of systemic, calcu-
lated, and intentional choices. I hope every classroom across the country
reads this book and I hope every harm reductionist embraces it. With its
publication, we finally have a book that represents us degenerates, drug
users, sex workers, queer people in a way that honors our experiences
and celebrates our wisdom."—**Zoe Odlin-Platz**, Director of Operations,
Church of Safe Injection

"*How to Break an Addiction* is brilliant, gutting, miraculous, uncategoriz-
able. It will crowbar-open neglected parts of your brain and set your heart
on fire. It is not so much a book about addiction or the opioid crisis, as a
book about our pain under capitalism and what it means to be an Earth-
ling. Annie Spencer guides us gently through the centuries, the science,
the Marxist theory, the contours of the precipice otherwise known as our
times in poetic prose that is easy to understand, that sings, that trans-
ports, that reminds us about the best aspects of ourselves, that we have
purpose and we have possibility."—**Owen Toews**, author of *Island Falls*
and *Stolen City: Racial Capitalism and the Making of Winnipeg*

"An essential corrective to overdetermined narratives of addiction that
locate the opioid crisis in either the damaged brains of users or in the
unscrupulous hands of doctors, dealers, and pharma reps, Annie Spencer
centers a capitalist logic that alienates us from forms of solidarity and
violently clears ground for extractive profit. Clear-eyed in their outrage
and grief, Spencer promiscuously moves between form, discipline and
context in this essential indictment of a global system that keeps us in
pain in order to sell us the fix."—**Benjamin Haber**, Assistant Professor of
Sociology, Wesleyan University

"As a mutual aid and harm reduction project committed to sharing resources and redistributing wealth throughout the Kensington community, we think *How to Break An Addiction* is essential reading for anyone involved in similar work. This book humanizes our community members through its analysis, compellingly arguing that addiction is not a moral failing but a failure of a society reliant on capitalism. Dr. Spencer expertly identifies the pernicious ways the capitalist mode of production accumulates wealth through dispossession, especially for those that capital must fail in order to grow."—**Community Action Relief Project**, a mutual aid organization in Philadelphia, PA

"This book isn't just a story about the so-called 'addict,' the demon drug of OxyContin, or, even, the most evil people in the pharmaceutical industry (meet the Sacklers!). It is, at its core, a crime story about capitalism: how capitalism makes addicts of all of us but how the true addict is capital itself; how this dead but dominant paradigm destroys personal lives, but also planetary life. Damning as it is, *How to Break an Addiction* is also deeply funny, generous, personal, moving—and, dare I say, healing! In short: this is *the* book about the opioid epidemic you want to hold in your hand to make sense of the world and the book you want holding your hand too as you break free."—**Mikkel Frantzen**, author of *Going Nowhere, Slow: The Aesthetics and Politics of Depression*

"We know that capitalism is about the reign of abstractions, of surplus value over life, of abstract labor over the laboring body. These abstractions are codified and reified in the discipline of economics, which abstract itself from the lives that are wrecked in the wake of the pursuit of profit. What would it mean to think concretely? How can we locate thought in our bodies, in our struggle, and this moment? Annie Xibos Spencer's *How to Break an Addiction: A Method-in-a-Manifesto for Quitting Capitalism* is not just a book on the opioid epidemic and its situation with late-capitalist strategies of exploitation and extraction, but a demonstration of how one can think in-and-through the specificity of one's situation, one's struggles, and even one's pain to produce a common strategy for struggle and liberation."—**Jason Read**, author of *The Double Shift: Spinoza and Marx on the Politics of Work*

"Annie Xibos Spencer, whose prose indicates that she could have just as likely been a rapper than a geographer, gives us a scholarly and accessible map of the people, policies, and corporations behind the opioid epidemic as well as our collective social pain. Our space-age materialist tour guide reveals the economic causes of chronic pain and morbidity and reveals that our recovery is predicated on a revolution that is more powerful than the chemicals. Substance users of the world, unite! We have nothing to lose but our chronic existential and physical pain!"—**Cassie Thornton**, author of *The Hologram: Feminist, Peer-to-Peer Health for a Post-Pandemic Future*

"Spencer's work is a tour de force that effortlessly moves between the personal and the structural and thereby evokes the best of critical theory while at the same time producing an altogether novel approach to the most pressing societal issues of our time."—**Björn Karlsson**, organizer and scholar activist, IT University of Copenhagen

"This beautiful, forcefully argued book wrestles our understanding of addiction away from pathology and punishment, placing it exactly where it must be: in a history of capital, an extractive economic system which is fundamentally against life. Across these pages, Spencer argues that if our social movements strive, on the other hand, to be for life, then we must without question be on the side of those who have been treated as disposable and discarded as 'addicts.' Far from a call to rescue people from drug use, *How To Break an Addiction* reveals that understanding the political economy of the opioid epidemic's devastation is a necessary step to saving ourselves from the death-making and deadening forces of capitalism today."—**Craig Willse**, author of *The Value of Homelessness*

"*How to Break an Addiction* is a stellar analysis on the unavoidable poisons in the framework of survival. The wiring of our consciousness, our access to wellness, and our cognitive ability to separate truth from trauma, deteriorates under capitalism, destroying our voice and our purpose. In *How to Break an Addiction*, studying the opioid epidemic becomes the axis between surviving systemic abuse and accessing self-care."—**Cristy Road Carrera**, author, artist; *Next World Tarot, Spit & Passion*

"The ongoing opioid 'epidemic' is a racialized class war. It is capitalism feeding on the misery it has created, presenting a gory scene full of murderous contradictions. What would an epic detective story read like if the victim were a whole society, if the killer were a system, and if the sleuth was not a cop but a comrade? This remarkable book offers us a model. It moves with precision, grace, and compassion between theory, testimony, political economy, history, biography, science, and vision. File it under a radical forensics, but rippling with a quiet, queer hope. It not only shows us the bodies, the motive, and the method of this monumental crime. Like the best of such stories, this one invites us to see the glint of solidarity in the grit and darkness, and by that light to find our way through the long night back to day."—**Max Haiven**, author of *Revenge Capitalism: The Ghosts of Empire, the Demons of Capital, and the Settling of Unpayable Debts*

HOW TO BREAK AN ADDICTION

HOW TO BREAK AN ADDICTION
A METHOD-IN-A-MANIFESTO FOR QUITTING CAPITALISM

Annie Xibos Spencer

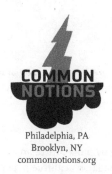

Philadelphia, PA
Brooklyn, NY
commonnotions.org

How To Break an Addiction:
A Method-in-a-Manifesto for Quitting Capitalism
© Annie Xibos Spencer

This edition © 2024 Common Notions

ISBN: 978-1-945335-19-8 | eBook ISBN: 978-1-945335-35-8
Library of Congress Number: 2024945585

10 9 8 7 6 5 4 3 2 1

Common Notions   Common Notions
c/o Interference Archive   c/o Making Worlds Bookstore
314 7th St.   210 S. 45th St.
Brooklyn, NY 11215   Philadelphia, PA 19104

www.commonnotions.org
info@commonnotions.org

Discounted bulk quantities of our books are available for organizing, educational, or fundraising purposes. Please contact Common Notions at the address above for more information.

Cover design by Josh MacPhee
Layout design and typesetting by Suba Murugan
Printed by union labor in Canada on acid-free paper

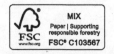

I can't be a pessimist because I'm alive.
—*James Baldwin*

For my family. For the species. For the planet. Let's get free.

CONTENTS

ACKNOWLEDGMENTS

A TOAST OF GRATITUDE

Making this book was almost the death of me and I'm not the only one.

Erika and Malav, Stella, Syd, Jeff and the rest of the workers at Common Notions Press—I owe you a debt of gratitude that stretches spacetimes and makes the kinds of ties that bind, in love and fire, in revolutionary times. Thank you from the bottom of my heart.

The completion of this book marks the end of some big cycle in my life. In a parafictional retelling, it's like I broke the world real bad in a past life and I had a cosmic debt to do some part to put it back together again in this lifetime. Thanks to the many who helped me arrive home, here and now. I will miss many of your names, I fear. But the connection remains. The gift lives on, multiplies, spreads like a virus.

I was lucky to have some friends who really helped me, saw me, and could make space for me while I was in a state of emergence that was not legible to most in ways that left me vulnerable to extinction. There were some key moments where people loved me actively by reaching back and helping me hold space for a major integration to unfold as me.

Gabriel Defazio, Ali Mann, Cassie Thornton, Kristen Gallagher, Magda Härtelova, Mariana Pinzón, Haga Frey, Viki Karato, Flupsi, Mikkel Krause Frantzen, Martin Sunnerdahl, Morgan Buck, Farhan Sarwar, Tianao Guo, Ivar Fersters, Ariel Avery, Azize Güneş, Jonathan Rochkind, and Katie Wallis in particular, gifted me a degree of stability, acceptance, and space to grow into myself. These people made an enormous and positive difference in a particularly crucial phase of my journey, between the summer 2020 and the completion of this text in the summer of 2024.

Many others helped me too with their friendship, comradery, and presence. Some of them are: Raymond Luc Levasseur, Ahmed Magdy

El-Gendy, Noemi Frenk, Marita Sunnerdahl, Florence Freitag, Ara Hacopian, Brett Story, Dolly-Rae Star, Sónia Vaz Borges, Christina Heatherton, Sally O'Neil, Sonya Collier, Ben Haber, Sharon Haber, Pilo Marimón, Cash Hauke, Glynis Hull-Rochelle, Jared Radding, Seth Baker, Bronwyn Dobchuk-Land, Owen Toews, Oskar Weinberger, Nils Brandsma, Isa Knafo, Steve McFarland, Hector Rivera, Anna Swisher, Zoe Odlin-Platz, Lizzy Garnatz, Christina Cook, Chris Bearclaw, Katie Keating, Caroline Teschke, Karine Odlin, Rob Korobkin, Sage Hayes Kareem Rabie, Michael Menser, Kandice Chuh, Ahmed Shamim, Anupam Das, Shibani Das, Farida Akther, Farhad Mazhar, Max Haiven, Leigh Claire La Berge, Neil Agarwal, Francesca Manning, Jeremy Umali, Laura Diewald, Samaa Abdurraqib, Rachel Goffe, Vinay Gidwani, Nick Underwood, Pujita Guha, Dory Cote, Jody Breton, John Moore, Michael Wilkerson, Debbie Wilkerson, Anna Wiberg, Anna Hernmar, Niklas Ekström, Martin Pettersson, Richard Öhman, Martin Andersson, Hilde Andersen, and Siv Hansson.

Thanks and love to my living brothers: Joseph, James, and Augustus. And to our departed brother, Michael Xibos.

Ideas are always co-creations and mine have mingled and been shaped and improved by countless others. In particular, by my comrades, colleagues, teachers, and friends at and affiliated with the CUNY Graduate Center, as well as those at George Washington University and New College of Florida. I'm also grateful to my students at the University of Southern Maine, Bates College, and Hunter College CUNY.

* * *

Thanks to the committees and collectives of rebellious thought that nurtured my intellectual curiosity and development in my time at the Grad Center: the Mellon Committee on Globalization and Social Change, the Center for Place, Culture and Politics, and the Spacetime Research Collective.

Thank you to the Hologram community of practice, the Berlin Hologram Gang, and the UGH Posse. Thank you for the space, possibility and expansion we make together. It transforms me again and again. ∞

Thanks to the internationalists, radicals, queers, organizers and underground culture world builders in Skåne and Øresund whose presence and activity makes space for my existence, my wellbeing, here. Thanks to the Repan gang and the Thursday jam crew. Thanks to the Christiania Sundhedshus collective.

Among the dearly departed, special thanks to:
Mary Xibos Spencer, Charles Spencer, Michael Xibos, Joseph Spencer, Daniel Spencer, Alex Xibos, Patrick Xibos, Annie Xibos Hoffman, Blanca Mantovani Underwood, David Zysk, Ilya Azbuki, Sadhan Das, Jesse Harvey, and Sue Houchins.

An extra word of gratitude to my extraordinary teachers:
David Harvey, Neil Smith (RIP), and Ruth Wilson Gilmore.

Sláinte, Skål, Cheers, *Salud, Yamas . . .*

In love and devotion,
Annie

INTRODUCTION

Fee-fee, fi-fi, fo-fo fum
I smell the blood of a million sons
A million daughters from a
Hundred thousand guns
Not taught by our teachers on
Our curriculum
Do you hear that thunder?
That's the sound of strength in numbers

—IDLES, "Grounds" (2017)

This book is about the opioid epidemic and is the culmination of what immersive, rigorous, multimodal study on and struggle with the opioid epidemic taught me about how we all get free. Capitalism cannot be reformed or regulated into being on the side of life. A viable future for humanity requires a postcapitalist revolution that begins with a collective consciousness shift. To that end, this book argues for a paradigm shift away from capitalism and its knowledge regime toward new and renewed ways of understanding, inquiring, problem solving, and provisioning.

The book jumps scales and timelines in an attempt to arrive at the present moment in enough depth and dimension to claim some *tierra firma* in common. I use the phrase "tierra firma"[1] (meaning "solid

---

1.   In the final act of writing this introduction, I want to provide some explanation about this book's use of Spanish phrases, like "tierra firma" as opposed to the more commonly used "terra firma." The phrases have come to me organically as organizing devices for my own thought process and theory making. One guess as to why is that an early, illuminating and

1

ground"), to hark back to capital's existential imperative for space, for territory to circulate through (affix to, transmute, and leave), in order to be realized as profits. Accumulation, the quest for ever-growing profit, is a spatial process. It is the Earth and her living, interrelated parts that hold value in the system. Seeing this fact ought to draw urgent scrutiny to the incongruence of exchange value and use value in capitalism. More often than not, this affixing and alchemizing process creates ruin in real terms, while only profit is recorded in the terms of the dead but dominant paradigm.

Dead but dominant paradigm is my name for the colonial knowledge system that partitions, reduces, isolates, and immobilizes the interdependent concert of life. It names and diagnoses the colonial knowledge regime. For most people from the Western world, training ourselves to see and diagnose the dead but dominant paradigm is akin to teaching a fish to do the same with water. In diagnosing the flattened, reductive, economistic paradigm dead but dominant, I echo Neil Smith's diagnosis of neoliberalism as dead but dominant in 2008.[2] More than signifying that it has "run its course," I also mean to call it lifeless. The paradigm of partition is the paradigm of plunder. The knowledge regime that runs the world today, with its carved-up, quantified abstractions, is running it into the ground. Revelations in medicine that see the interrelatedness of the *body and mind* as an integral, relational system—the *bodymind* or the *soma*—or studies of the global mycelial network (called "the circulatory system of the planet") are but a few emerging harbingers of the paradigm shift in the making, away from abstraction and dualism toward relational, dynamic, and multidimensional kinds of understanding and inquiry. A collective consciousness rooted in relational understanding is necessary for producing economic policy that remembers, acknowledges, and reveres what it is to be human together on a living Earth.

Golpe growth is a phrase I use to convey the commonality within capitalism of grand seizures through concerted acts of violence. *Golpe* is a Spanish word meaning "a blow or a bang." A *coup d'etat* is

---

formative experience of thinking about global processes and structures and how to change the world occurred for me when I was studying global political economy in Spanish-language-conducted courses in Buenos Aires in 2002.

2.   Neil Smith, "Comment: Neoliberalism: Dominant but Dead," *Focaal* 51 (August 2008): 155–157.

a *golpe de estado*. I heard the word a lot while I was living in Argentina amidst the economic crisis in 2002 and studying Latin American political economy. I use the term to convey that coups, invasions, large-scale theft, hostile takeovers and other kinds of what gets called "so-called primitive accumulation" in Marx's work, or "accumulation by dispossession" or supposedly "extra-economic means" by David Harvey and other Marxist theorists, is ordinary, baked into the capitalist mode of production, a part of the thing, not an exception or an outlier to it. I use golpe growth as a consciousness device, to give a name that evokes a history of how this system actually works, how it stays afloat, all it must continually tear asunder. So-called primitive accumulation is ongoing and an essential feature of capitalism, conveniently left out of the colonial knowledge system's paradigm of economic theory and modeling, where students waste their lifeforce so neatly graphing price-quantity dynamics with rulers and pencils. Rosa Luxemburg, Maria Mies, and Farida Akhter, among others, taught me to see it and to direct my curiosity, to theorize, into the space of its erasure.

Meaning-making, map-making, future-making, is all part and parcel to the work of charting a course from here and now to something better that we imagine into being together. Imagining-into-being is another way to conceive of organizing, planning, and collective decision making. By linking theory, experience, evidence, and history, the work aims to help us to better recognize and make meaning from circumstances comprising the present, to read the signs of the times in a way that renders visible available channels, pathways, streams, and bridges by which we might produce a peaceful and abundant future for humanity and life on Earth.

In an attempt to break free from the system's engrained patterning and stuck loops, the book jumps tracks, creating openings. The political project of creating space is the work of creating possibility. Into that space we might assert agency, conduct the available energy already in motion with intention, presence, and renewed kinds of collective action. The chapters of the book operate as an eight-pronged spiral. Starting with the opioid epidemic in focus, I turn the kaleidoscope a notch and tell a related story from a different angle, creating more dimensions of our interrelated field, attuning more collective consciousness. The intention is to offer a toolkit for traversing the *present in crisis*, to offer a way of seeing, knowing, researching, and waging revolution.

The book examines the devastation capital brings at different scales: to the body, the social body, and the living Earth. It is deft at changing its story; it shifts shape. Seeing capital in process and across different dimensions is key to breaking free from the many ways it colonizes our minds and partitions our capacity to adequately see or diagnose what needs changing. Onto the partition wall, the system projects stories (white lies, historiographies) about why things are the way they are. These stories, which are not the truth, are used to justify why we don't live in a more beautiful world. They're used to explain away preventable harm and to incapacitate or placate us, to discourage us from seeing ourselves in one another, and from seeing ourselves as agents of revolutionary change. They're also used to manipulate us into fighting in or rooting for the endless stream of wars that the capitalist system cannot live without. Partitioned consciousness and the stories projected onto the fourth wall are meant to throw us off course from our species' innate curiosity and desire to make creative improvements. It confuses our sense of what is and is real (ontology), how it came to be that way (conflating the real facts of history with historiography), what can be studied (epistemology) and what is to be done (ideology). This is to say nothing of all the harm the colonial knowledge regime has done to our capacity to remember our place in a living universe, our sense of what it's worth, what's possible, and what we're here for (faith). I call this essential severing *the departure from the real*.

METHOD IN A MANIFESTO

The line of inquiry that unfolds in the book demonstrates what Bertell Ollman calls the "dance of the dialectic."[3] For me, this is a practice of somatic scholarship. In order to answer my questions—about where here and now is—I had to come home to myself, to suture together a fragmented consciousness, to learn to inhabit my body, to find a

---

3. Bertell Ollman, *Dance of the Dialectic: Steps in Marx's Method* (Champaign: University of Illinois Press, 2003).

way to *be* in the here and now. Recovery required me to put my whole being into the inquiry, to recover from the colonial education system's disembodiment, domination, and discipline.

I hope to demonstrate a model of inquiry that can be replicated. I hope to model how to follow the money to undo the world. I hope to exemplify how healing, done well, makes us a threat to the existing dis-order of things; how to honor our stories, our body knowledge, and our ancestral lived experience to create the world where we belong, all things in common. There's joy in this method. I hope to inspire relational scholarship, where we learn, create, question and revise, together.

Chapter 1, "Everyday Life in Permanent Crisis," introduces me, the opioid epidemic, and the context and tenor of the text. I began studying the opioid epidemic for my doctoral dissertation research, while in a state of embodied, material crisis. The chapter frames and substantiates my enduring question: how might I, we, survive this impasse?

Chapter 2, "Teaching Economics at the End of the Paradigm," takes aim at the dead but dominant knowledge system by relaying some of my experience as Visiting Assistant Professor in Macroeconomics at the University of Southern Maine in 2018–2019. It attempts to render obvious the connection between the intellectual paucity of the discipline of economics and the present's proliferation of crises, including endless warfare and "addiction." Traversing an American landscape of late-neoliberal humanitarian crisis, I demonstrate that the flattened and lifeless paradigm, with its fetish of two-dimensional, price-quantity modeling, displaces the onus of harm, leaves us busy with bare-life survival and insufficiently equipped to orient ourselves toward life-giving and meaningful change.

Chapter 3, "Finding a Fix," makes the case for understanding the opioid epidemic as a byproduct of the neoliberal turn. I show how breaking the backs of the American blue-collar working class—coupled with the intensification of debt, warfare, and carceral regimes of unfreedom—created the possibility for this massive foreclosure of life. I demonstrate how the capture of institutions of knowledge production and governance by the capitalist class churned laboring and would-be-laboring people into tierra firma. Like other kinds of resurgent extractivism, with the opioid epidemic, people's living bodies became conduits for cashing out profits. By getting people hooked, white and black market narcocapitalists get the fix they need, ever-higher returns on investment.

Chapter 4, "What of the Addict?" reframes the common-sense notion of addiction as a personal problem, offering instead a relational, material, psycho-spiritual understanding. Destigmatizing and depathologizing the condition of disordered consumption, the chapter reframes the question of dependency, diagnosing the disordered social order as what's sick and needs changing. It also shows how the racial capitalist state justifies the necessary group-differentiated partitions of status, stigma, privilege, and punishment that are essential to the system's maintenance.

In Chapter 5, "Capital is a Fiend," we travel spacetime with the morphine molecule, in order to show commonalities between the present moment and earlier, imperial phases of accumulation. It helps us understand the long history and present-day articulations of colonial, racial capitalism. The chapter examines the British-Chinese Opium Wars and makes the case for understanding drugs as bedrock financial assets, even as currency.

Chapter 6, "Tramps Like Us," is a materialist memoir told in place-based vignettes. It is an exercise in somatic inquiry, of naming some of the specters that haunted the research. It gives some context for understanding the lived experience of the American blue-collar working class in decline, on the run, facing precipitating conditions of foreclosure, confinement, and unfreedom.

Chapter 7, "Addiction as an Accumulation Strategy," demonstrates that the opioid epidemic repeats an observable pattern in which a crisis that is produced in accordance with capital's logic becomes a new revenue stream for the creation of further profits, thus creating further crisis. It demonstrates that resolving the harms produced by capitalism can only be done with a new and socially accountable system. It shows that capital cannot be regulated, tamed, or defanged and argues that it instead must be transcended, overcome, with a consciousness shift that allows us to see it as it shifts shape, to be wiser than its narratives of help or goodness of fit.

Chapter 8, "Bodies in Revolt," offers provocations on the connection between the epidemic of chronic physical pain that launched the opioid epidemic and the rise of right-wing political formations in the

US. The appeal of fascism is that it offers an explanatory framework that coopts an existing sentiment of rage, alienation, and resentment.

BREAKING AN ADDICTION

Breaking an addiction doesn't have to mean sobriety or abstinence. It means no longer using in an extractive or auto-extractive way, no longer feeling like we need to go too hard in any direction, consumptive or otherwise, to get by. Enhancing our wellbeing, pursuing our heart's true desire—not seeking escape or oblivion—becomes our guiding principle. It is the coming into a supportive network of life in community, in context, that allows us to expand our time horizon, not needing to focus on coping, obtaining the next short-term fix for all that feels unlivable, unmanageable, painful, or frightening.

A huge and under-addressed part of the problem of so-called addiction is that human beings behave irrationally. We act against our stated will and in allegiance with distorted fantasies and powerful fears that cloud our consciousness—including our understanding of who we are, what life is for, and what we might otherwise be capable of creating together. This is a fact of humanity: the psychosocial phenomenon of disordered, commodity comfort-seeking rests on a bedrock of violence, an accumulation of the horrors of history.

Capitalism is against life itself to its very core. Marx and Engels rightly foretold nearly two centuries ago that the system contained the seeds of its own destruction, that it would collapse under the weight of its own internal contradictions, most evident among them—its insatiable quest for *more* on a planet with finite resources. They were too optimistic about humans' capacity to *see* beyond it; perhaps they could not account for the innovation in mind games, illusions, and mental trickery.

In a profit-centric world dis-order, every scientific advancement on how human beings work is put to work first and fastest on the quest to keep us on the system's hook. Capitalism and its state and quasi-state formations wage war against our capacity to recognize ourselves in one another and see each other as parts of an integral whole. Technologies of partition allow the system and its actors to wage ongoing war on life itself. These innovations in division, divisiveness, disappearing, and destruction proliferate the capacity to shape and distort what is on our minds, what we think and what we think we know.

On the verge of collapse, the system's agents now seek its preferred form of reset—world war and its others, catastrophic calamity born of climate collapse, rising cartel formations, land grabs, and other kinds of *golpes*. History tells us, when capital cannot find a profitable means to reinvestment, it settles for creative destruction. Through overt and covert financing maneuvers, capitalists line up to bet on the one left standing atop the rubble pile with the most important thing a capitalist facing crisis can imagine: a clean slate to begin accumulating again.

BECOMING ECOSYSTEMIC

Becoming ecosystemic is the process (the road we make by walking) of summoning into being in the material realm that which we know we have the capacity to create otherwise. Becoming ecosystemic means returning to the senses, and to the perceptive intelligence of the soma that feels and knows our interconnectedness with all beings. This is the true insight of the quantum turn in theoretical physics: there are no disentangled discrete parts; all parts are parts to a whole that define and are defined by said whole. This concept is also at the crux of dialectical thinking.

The opioid epidemic began primarily as a "white" and "suburban" and "rural" phenomenon, but has touched the lives of Americans from all racial and ethnic backgrounds. This book dislodges "whiteness" as a frame of reference to illuminate the workings of racial capitalism; how racial order and structural domination is made and remade in shifting regimes of economic accumulation. Following Cedric Robinson, the book uses an analytical framework that understands that all capitalism is racial capitalism. Capitalism is addicted to warfare. The book teaches us to see this fact up close, from a vantage informed by a political and intellectual legacy on which to lean while we do the work of decolonizing, which includes a lot of unraveling, letting go, grieving, beginning again. This method offers an analogy to the recovery from substance dependence. We harvest the lessons and wisdom of the path toward a nonaddictive, nonextractive way of living and being together. Becoming ecosystemic is the consciousness shift of living

revolution, leading with our felt senses and knowing our interconnectedness, arriving home, already whole.

A NOTE ON LANGUAGE AND CONCEPTS

Why I don't call people "addicts."
The history of the word is saturated in stigma and shame, as elaborated in Chapter 4. The word often obscures both the mechanisms at play in a complex social health phenomenon as well as taking focus off the locus of harm, a society based on irrational consumption and that promotes one thing above all—dependency that deteriorates.

Why I'm sparing with the word "addiction."
Plenty has been said about the continuum of consumption-based coping mechanisms. In an era where the medicalized "brain disease" model of so-called addiction is resurgent, the term can be used to pathologize certain means of ritualized comfort-seeking while obscuring the continuity of drug taking with other more socially acceptable or even rewarded habits, like workaholism or what I call "wealth-accumulation disorder."

Why I'm sparing with "substance use disorder."
I find the neologism a huge improvement over "addiction," and am in solidarity with the movements who advocate for drug users with an insistence on this change in language. I find the concept, as part and parcel of the medical model of addiction presently in vogue with major funding institutions and research design, overemphasizes the individual's physiology.

Why I don't say "abuse."
This word has a charge to it that refers to criminality and violence. Recall that in Nixon's press conference announcing a new campaign against America's "public enemy number one," he named that enemy *drug abuse*. The official record shows the maneuver was a tactic to ensnarl and repress left liberation movements. Abuse suggests pathology, immorality, and a threat to common decency. To me, the word "abuse" in the context of drug taking or dependency is sensational and politically productive of social harm against people who use drugs. As a language device, abuse serves to dislocate the onus of harm done.

Why I don't say "clean."
To call people who abstain from substances *clean* is to imply that people who use substances are *dirty*. We are not.

*Why I don't say "j**kie."*
In my estimation, this word belongs to the category of words that are only rightly used by people who have had said word used against them as a weapon intending to dehumanize.

Why I don't say "relapse."
Making healthy changes is hard. Breaking old habits is tricky. Humans have free will and we also have an unconscious. Relapse suggests failure and finality. Often the narrative of a relapse implies that one trying to make life-affirming changes is 'right back where they started,' which is never the case. As long as we live another day, we're still in the game, and that in itself is progress. Trying is holy. Trying and failing is sacred. Trying and failing and trying again? Now that's truly living.

CHAPTER 1

EVERYDAY LIFE IN PERMANENT CRISIS

Take a moment and look around to the people standing beside you—
maybe you know them, maybe you don't. Exchange a glance with
them; introduce yourselves to each other. Appreciate this moment;
appreciate their aliveness; appreciate their humanity; appreciate
your own compassion. Allow for the collective grief that is among
us tonight to weigh heavy on your hearts and also appreciate that.

—David Zysk, opening remarks, Overdose Awareness March and Vigil,
Portland, Maine, August 31, 2015

On September 1, 2015, I awoke at my apartment in Portland, Maine,
made a cup of coffee, and checked the state and local news coverage
of an event I had helped organize the previous evening—the second
annual march and public vigil for the rising drug overdose deaths
in my community and nationwide. The event, to which a few hundred people had come, comprised a march past City Hall, down Preble Street, where the huge homeless services nonprofit by the same
name sits, continued beyond the library and the city-owned Oxford
Street homeless shelter, and led back to Monument Square, where we
took our places under the Portland Sailors and Soldiers Monument,
an American Civil War tribute dedicated in 1891. In the company of
a large bronze statue of a goddess with sword and shield, Our Lady
of Victories, we gathered for a candlelight vigil, remarks from invited
speakers, and an open-mic, open-air community share.

While looking through the photo gallery from the event on the
Bangor Daily News site, I got a phone call from my brother Jim in
Florida informing me that our brother Joe had overdosed and been

hospitalized for a second time in the span of a few days. After the first incident, I phoned the hospital's nurses and administrators, pleading with them not to release him until there was space available for him in an accessible (free) detox or rehab facility. Joe was scheduled to turn himself in at the county courthouse later that week to serve another jail sentence, this time for nine months, and I sensed that Joe's overdose was in some way an expression of his will not to return to living in a cage, where he'd already spent a combined year and a half. A sensitive person by nature, among the stories he'd shared with me about his time inside, the features he remembered with a shudder included the constant high-decibel noise (people screaming angrily for different reasons, mentally broken people constantly chattering and emoting, and a ceaseless cell-block-wide contest to make the most thunderous GONG sound by hurling an object of one's choosing at the cell-standard, metal toilet bowl) and the lights—stark halogens that buzz and flicker and never shut off or even dim for sleeping. But alas, with no beds for the "indigent" at any of the local facilities, and with no medical or legal reason to warrant holding him, he was released. This time, Jim said, Joe was in a coma, his kidneys showed signs of failure, and I should consider making plans to get there.

I was scheduled to work a volunteer shift at the Needle Exchange Program of the now-defunct India Street Public Health Clinic, and set out by foot, not wanting to be anywhere else in the moment than with the community of practitioners and clients I had grown close with there, who understood the overwhelming and relentless shock and grief associated with this crisis, and who taught me a lot in my year and a half of once-or twice-weekly volunteering, about finding my own capacity to show up amidst it. Some of my favorite exchange members came in that day, including a few who had helped put the previous night's event together or had movingly spoken at it. In my conversations with staff and members, we all agreed the event was a success, and expressed our gratitude that rather than the "scared-straight" moralism we were worried might blow over from the segments of the local sober community that were actively hostile to harm reductionism, the overwhelming message of the evening was about our shared humanity amidst unspeakable shared pain. Despite marching in the streets behind a banner that read "Not One More!"—the tone of the speaking and vigil portion felt more like a ritual of public mourning than a demonstration. The co-organizers and attendees I spoke with throughout the day all felt that making space and time for acknowledging, feeling, and gathering amidst the crisis was some unspoken prerequisite to any meaningful mass action.

I was finishing an exchange with a baby-faced, thirty-six-year-old man (notable because, in my observations, injection drug use ages people prematurely) when I heard an urgent banging on the exchange door and screaming coming from the other side. I was careful not to rush while the desperate knocking and moaning continued. When he'd readied himself to exit, we exchanged knowing nods about needing to be braced for whatever situation was unfolding on the other side of the door.

I opened the door to a scraggly-haired, thin man with swollen and calloused hands I so commonly saw among The Exchange's clients, the hands of laboring and once-laboring people. When my mother came to visit me in 2009, when I lived in New York City, she was nearly totally wheelchair bound. My then-partner and I took her and my father on a car tour of Manhattan in our 1991 Toyota Camry station wagon. She spent the whole ride looking straight up and remarking about the *hands*, the *human hands*, the *laboring-men's hands*, that constructed the feats that dazzled our eyes, confounded, entertained, and housed us. This man with laboring hands before me now looked to be about fifty years old.

He was sweating, pacing, and weak-kneed: *"My brother, oh God, my brother!* You gotta help me! He's OUT; He's *OUT!"*

Bob, I would learn, moaned and shouted. I asked if he needed Narcan, the overdose reversal drug that was still hard to access in Maine, but for which The Exchange had been receiving rogue shipments from a harm reduction organization elsewhere in the country, an illegal act that could have jeopardized their nonprofit status, or the India Street Clinic's city charter, but which they did regularly. The Exchange had been giving out Narcan for a year at that point, and opioid and heroin users throughout Southern Maine knew of us, if not because they exchanged dirty-for-clean works with us, then because they or someone they know had an overdose reversed with one of our Narcan kits. That Bob drove his brother to the India Street Clinic, and not to the hospital, is telling. He knew we could help him and that needing our help wouldn't get him punished the way a trip to the ER likely would in the absence of a state "Good Samaritan" law. I yelled a heads-up to the staff and headed outside with Bob and two of the kits that volunteers and staff were always readying during downtime, containing two tiny, glass vials of naloxone, an alcohol swab, rubber gloves, and two intramuscular syringes. We found his brother, glistening with a light sweat, blue, and lifeless in the front seat of a gold, early 1990s American sedan, and I popped the orange plastic cap on the vial and drew up the first syringe, laser focused, adrenaline-driven, and steadying my hands. By then, some clinical staff members had caught up with us. A nurse named Michelle exposed and prepared the man's chest with the alcohol swab, while I gladly passed the naloxone preparation to the clinic's physician, Dr. Ann Lemire, for the immediate next task of injecting Bob's brother.

Bob's brother took his first gasp for air right as the police and an ambulance were arriving. With the medical team tending to the patient, a staff person named Elisabeth and I turned our attention back to Bob, who was still in shock. Instinctively, I knew he needed to be brought into the present moment, out of his solitary, severed fright, and into the relational field. "You did the right thing, Bob. He's alive, look; he's breathing. You saved your brother's life, Bob. You're both going to be okay." It was my best attempt at a "trauma-informed standard of care," otherwise known as comradely compassion. When supporting someone coming out of shock, it is best to create a container of presence. Attempting nervous system coregulation, orient them to what has happened, and provide convincing assurance of their capacity to survive it. This is attuned presence, a most essential tool in the revolutionary toolkit. It is kryptonite to alienation. See how it tracks with your ancestors' stories of survival.

The police officers interrupted us to ask what had transpired before their arrival. They were bothered, procedural, and condescending. With Bob's brother secured to a stretcher being hoisted into the ambulance and the driver of the car being taken into handcuffs, a young patrolman emerged from the car with a dirty tin and unfinished deck [bag of heroin] and, while wearing a smirk, attempted to joke with the officers and clinic personnel. "If you're going to be a junkie, you'd think you'd learn what fentanyl looks like!" He looked to us for an affirmation, apparently not noticing the difference in our affective states. I'm the child of blue-collar Scorpios. I react. "When did *you* learn what fentanyl looks like? Three weeks ago?" I found myself spitting back. "I guess it makes the job easier to do if you can pretend the people suffering in your midst aren't actually *people*," I managed to say. Noticing the O-mouthed-emoji faces of my Exchange comrades, I set out on an adrenaline-soaked walk around the block before returning to the clinic to finish the rest of my shift.

With data-driven hindsight, this day occurred amid a dramatic spike in overdoses as fentanyl and its analogues, between a hundred and a thousand times more potent than heroin, began showing up in the white-powder heroin and counterfeit pressed pills supply chain in the US. Opioid-dependent people sourcing their daily fix from the illicit supply chain were dying in droves. Even veteran heroin users— elders in the scene, around for decades, who taught newer users how to use safely—were falling. The cheaper, more compact, and readily available opioids came mostly from Canadian and Chinese labs at the time. They made their way to Maine via New York City or the port towns of Massachusetts.

In addition to the logistical cost-savings of its compactness, fentanyl emerges as the no-brainer technological adaptation, a so-called "labor-saving" innovation, of the heroin market. In 2019 even the "nonprofit" warfare economy "think tank" RAND Corporation, in their explainer on the rise of fentanyl, focused on the real driver of change: the logic of profit maximizing; not *demand*, as we're always told, but *supply-side* factors. Heroin must be grown in a field, in particular highland climates. It is subject to the whims of increasingly unpredictable weather patterns and harvested in a labor-intensive process that hasn't yet been mechanized. Fentanyl, on the other hand, is synthesized in a lab, meaning the inputs can be controlled. Once the initial investment has been made in the lab equipment and brick-and-mortar production facility, really only one worker, the chemist, is required in the production process. You've seen *Breaking Bad*?

In Volume I of *Capital*, Marx explains how the profit motive leads bakers to substitute some of the flour used in breadmaking with less costly ingredients, to keep the profit margins up. The drug trade, and all licit and illicit markets, operate according to this same capitalist logic, a compulsion to extract ever-growing profits by some manner of intensification in either the production process or the consumption circuitry. A coffee can of fentanyl packs the same high-inducing punch as a shipping container full of heroin. The introduction of fentanyl wasn't the result of *evil doers doing evil* but rather a predictable—rational, logical—outcome of a world order structured in capital's image. *Better, cheaper, faster.* Portland, Maine, a city of about 67,000 people, would see more than twenty-five police-involved overdose responses that week in September 2015, suggesting perhaps double that number went unreported to the police, for obvious reasons.

My involvement with the needle exchange was mutual-aid work. In the face of paralyzing fear, grief and pain, a wise friend and fellow activist named Samaa gave it to me straight, telling me: "You need to make yourself useful to people whose circumstances are worse than yours." She was right. I needed to move the energy of my stuck feelings out of my body, to channel my rage and powerlessness into something beautiful. With my hands, putting together naloxone kits, and with my body and my presence, in the exchange room and in the streets, and with my voice, in Portland's City Hall and in the press, I began to finally feel solidarity, which I believe to be the antidote to alienation.

Simultaneously, I was researching and writing a dissertation on the opioid epidemic for a PhD in Geography from the City University of New York (CUNY) Graduate Center. I researched and wrote endlessly, in a fury, in stream-of-conscious purges, mostly not thinking of the end goal—becoming Dr. Spencer. The dialectically unfolding scholarly inquiry melded with my cognitive, embodied, social, and material state of emergency. I pursued my research questions with the fever of someone whose life was on the line. I researched, annotated, and wrote like I was defusing a bomb or maybe learning to assemble one. I was learning to master what Amílcar Cabral called "the weapon of theory."[1]

In his opening remarks at the march and vigil in Portland, David Zysk, an opioid epidemic activist and person in recovery, opened with a quote from Wendell Berry: "We need drugs, apparently, because we

---

1. Amílcar Cabral, "The Weapon of Theory," Address delivered to the first Tricontinental Conference of the Peoples of Asia, Africa and Latin America, Havana, Cuba, January 1966, https://www.marxists.org/subject/africa/cabral/1966/weapon-theory.htm.

have lost each other."[2] Having been raised by people who used substances to soften the edges of their own spiraling decline into isolation, compounding traumas and economic ruin, the words struck me as immediately true. Looking around at the crowd, I saw that others felt this same recognition in Berry's words. Alienation, dislocation, and hopelessness are epidemic in the current moment, but by the very definition of these feeling states, they feel personal and individuating, and thus remain insufficiently articulated and recognizable as a collective critique.

Neoliberal economic restructuring fed working-class Americans through the meat grinder of newly financialized regimes of capital accumulation. We were the class of people who labored with our hands, our bodies, our hearts. As these jobs were automated, outsourced, offshored and otherwise degraded, I watched my four older brothers come of age into a world order and in a country that no longer needed them, no longer valued them, and no longer had a place for them, except in its ever-expanding prison system or a crematorium.

I decided to pursue a PhD in 2010 as a survival strategy, when my previous survival strategies seemed to no longer suffice. I began working at fourteen. The youngest of five, I was the first to attend college, and between working, scholarships and loans, I put myself through my BA and MA. Growing up without enough of the stuff, in Ronald Reagan's America, I was quite convinced that money made the world go round and so in school, I studied economics and I followed the money. I sought answers to questions about inequality, poverty, debt, dispossession, and developmentalist schemes.

Aside from my own lived experience, I studied localized articulations of these global calamities in Argentina and Bangladesh. As my questioning grew deeper, I found myself bumping up against the dead but dominant thought paradigm—the colonial knowledge system that structures the world in disarray, with its quantitative, reductive abstractions divorced from tierra-firma–based relational implications. For example, while studying the Argentine Peso Crisis of 2001, economic authorities offered technical, objective-sounding explanations for the crisis that struck me as peculiar, essentially arguing that the

---

2.   Wendell Berry, *The Art of the Commonplace: The Agrarian Essays of Wendell Berry*, ed. Norman Wirzba (Washington, DC: Counterpoint, 2003).

real problem with the dollar-to-peso pegged exchange rate plan was that wages there are "sticky downward," which is a cute way of saying that union power and working-class consciousness made it harder than expected to force lower wages on the masses. Economics, like the dominant medical system, is full of these kinds of diagnoses that act as barriers to actually illuminating lines of inquiry. It was reading David Harvey's *Spaces of Global Capitalism* in my first summer in Dhaka, in 2007, that introduced me to the field of critical economic geography, where, to paraphrase Ruth Wilson Gilmore, we remember that edges are also interfaces.

Soon after finishing my master's in International Trade and Investment Policy from George Washington University, my body began refusing to do the high-stress policy jobs I had worked hard to qualify myself to do, and ultimately, that I needed to do in order to repay my student loans. I laid down for a nap after 6 a.m. yoga one morning at my apartment in the East Village, intending to get to the office later than usual but before 9 a.m., and stayed in bed for nearly a month. It was the beginning of a long unravelling.

A nervous system in a constant state of distress propelled me forward for more than thirty years. Always on high alert, my system lived as if keeping me one step ahead of the tiger it believed to be chasing me my whole life. My system's new strategy was instead to play possum, throwing me into whole-body chronic pain among other debilitating symptoms that were eventually called "autoimmune disorders." In the absence of a welfare state, entering a PhD program was a survival strategy, a way to take a respite from the working world, to have health insurance and my student loans in "remission," and enough money for food and rent.

As sociologist Jennifer M. Silva put it in her 2013 book *Coming Up Short: Working-Class Adulthood in an Age of Uncertainty*, I was navigating a present that was unmanageable and working toward a future that was increasingly unimaginable. This is to say nothing of the past, which, in all people living with untreated complex trauma, is very much present. I had initially planned to conduct my dissertation research on an anticapitalist feminist agrarian movement I had encountered in Bangladesh, but with catastrophe on the rise in my family of origin, and with the rebellion in my bodymind ramping up, I felt called to turn the lens on my own predicament. I switched gears and studied the same set of questions about survival, dispossession, structural violence, and liberation *much* closer to home.

LOCATING THE CRISIS: RELATIONAL SEEING AND KNOWING

Geographers study why what is happening happens where it does.

What is happening: extreme and chronic physical pain.
Location: my body; the bodies of one third of all Americans.[3]

What is happening: precipitous deterioration of life circumstances and possible futures.
Location: me, my family, and people "like us," most other Americans, most other people and lifeforms on Earth.

Now it's common knowledge, but at the time of my dissertation proposal defense, in February 2015, I needed to make the case to some of my committee members that the crisis I planned to study—an epidemic of dependence, social and premature death from pain and pain pills—was even happening. By this point, I had lost my brother Michael to what hadn't yet been coined a *"death of despair,"* and my brother Joe and my mother to the *social death* of active opioid dependence. My mother was prescribed and became dependent on opioids in 1993, when I was twelve years old. She was ahead of the trend, which tips in 1996, in the early dawn of NAFTA and following the FDA approval of OxyContin in December 1995 and its subsequent aggressive marketing for severe chronic, non-terminal-illness related pain.[4]

I'd seen senior citizen neighbors and family friends raise young grandchildren after their adult children died or were incarcerated for violations related to their drug habit. I'd supported two friends who had lost brothers to overdose deaths. I'd watched the woods behind my parents' house be bulldozed and turned into a strip mall that housed a pain management clinic, a Social Security office, a large

3.   Institute of Medicine (US) Committee on Advancing Pain Research, Care, and Education, *Relieving Pain in America: A Blueprint for Transforming Prevention, Care, Education, and Research* (Washington, DC: National Academies Press, 2011), https://www.ncbi.nlm.nih.gov/books/NBK92510/.
4.   Art Van Zee, "The Promotion and Marketing of OxyContin: Commercial Triumph, Public Health Tragedy," *American Journal of Public Health* 99, no. 2 (February 2009): 221–227; Sam Quinones, *Dreamland: The True Tale of America's Opiate Epidemic* (New York: Bloomsbury Press, 2016).

chain pharmacy, and a rent-to-own furniture store. I'd seen people pay for their month's supply of brand-name blood pressure medication or an unanticipated car repair by selling off some of their pain medication. I'd noticed that a milligram of oxycodone corresponded in street value, exactly to the value of a dollar, a 5 mg pill cost five bucks; an 80 mg pill, eighty bucks. I'd known about the cold-water extraction process for separating out the acetaminophen from a hydrocodone tablet long before I heard Kendrick Lamar rap about it on his 2011 release "A.D.H.D." I'd seen up close the grim psycho-socio, embodied economic landscapes of the "OxyContin Blues" before Steve Earle sang of its grip in Appalachia in 2007.

More than seeing the pills used to quell chronic pain, or merely to "get high," I'd seen pain pills used to numb the emotional devastation of foreclosure, job loss, bankruptcy, the death of a child deployed to forgotten-about wars in Iraq or Afghanistan, and other manifestations of grief, powerlessness, isolation, injustice, and rage for which there was no healthy outlet, no public conversation, and, most palpable and politically urgent by my estimations—no available language. In the supposed good old days of Obama, when the college educated felt the world to be shrinking and their opportunities expanding, I saw pain pills and heroin, eventually fentanyl, quell the pain of losing one's connections to place and purpose, to the present and to a possible future, as the blue-collar working class' structural abandonment was cast as personal failure, anomalous shitty luck, or evidence of depravity. But I mentioned none of this experience, this knowing, in my professional academic setting at my proposal defense. I simply tried to find the right waves to surf on the gulf that separated this knowing from what even critical economic geography might allow me to learn and teach about it.

My undergraduate economics professor at New College of Florida, Fred Strobel, used to say, "the plural of anecdote is not data," and yet increasingly we live in a world replete with perfectly foreseeable problems from practically anyone's vantage, that *the data*, or rather the experts who produce it as sound and sanctified, suggest we can ignore to the point of oblivion. The infrastructure, the metrics, the tools, the premises, and presumptions are not set up to help us answer questions about life on Earth; they are intended only to find an available path for capital to blaze in pursuit of its continuous circulation, valorization, and augmentation. Physicist and philosopher Thomas Kuhn spoke of this disconnect between knowledge and data, between evidence and observation, between what is and what can be said by way of explanation, in his 1962 *The Structure of Scientific Revolutions*. In short, when the sum and like character of supposed anomalies, externalities, or outliers burst the boundaries of a given paradigm's available mode of explanation, when that which breaks the mold cannot be explained away as incidental but suggests the inadequacy of the existing mold—this belies the need for a new way of seeing and knowing. Paradigm shifts, like all revolutions, happen both incrementally and in quantum leaps.

I set out to understand the opioid epidemic in the United States because the drugs played a central role in the ravaging of my family of origin. My methodology was survival by any means necessary. I churned over the evidence and the logics by which the foreclosure of life chances for myself, my kin, and the collective was produced as normal, natural, or inevitable—the result of bad choices and poor luck. I obsessed over the pieces of the puzzle that animated the slow violence of everyday American life that goes on with our apparent consent at the same time as it feeds on, extracts, and profits from the decimation of our life force in spacetimes from the embodied-mental-molecular to the galactic. In short, I learned that resolving the problem sufficiently requires systems-wide change. Before we mark the loss of life that comprises the ongoing crisis, let's briefly introduce the dependency-inducing substance in question.

PAPAVER SOMNIFERUM: A FLOWER FOR (FORCED) FORGETTING

Heroin, like morphine, is an opiate, meaning it is derived from opium and the opium poppy, *Papaver somniferum*, grown in the Earth's soil, while opioids—like brand-name OxyContin, Percocet, and other branded and generic formulations of oxycodone, hydrocodone, codeine and fentanyl, among other pharmaceutical variations—are synthetic derivatives of the morphine molecule that are wholly synthesized in a lab.[5] Opioids and opiates induce deep breathing, something craved by every stressed organism, and have for centuries been prescribed for respiratory ailments. Opiates appear in ancient and contemporary remedies for coughs and chest colds. Heroin has a long life as an explicit antidote against fear. This is what inspired its naming in a Bayer Pharmaceuticals laboratory in 1898: the drug's capacity to promote heroism, or at least blunt all sensations relating to fear and its relatives, pain, grief, and despair.

The opium poppy is among the first and most widely used medicinal plants in human history. While preserved seeds and pods have been found in Neolithic Swiss artifacts from 4000 BC, it is widely believed that the opium poppy originates from lower Mesopotamia. Archaeological records dating to 3400 BC indicate that the Sumerians called the flower *Hul Gil*, or Joy Plant. Sumerians transferred the plant and knowledge of the cultivation of opium, the sap produced from lashing the pod of the flower, to the Assyrians, who spread it to the Babylonians, and they to the Egyptians. Egyptian cultivation and trading increased the plant's reach, popularity, and profitability. By 1400 BC the opium poppy had spread to points along the Phoenician trade routes of the era including North Africa, Asia Minor, Greece, and points in Europe. Archaeologists have found cultivation and harvest instruments dating from 1400 BC in Cyprus. While ancient Greek and Roman societies possessed the plant, and records and literature document its common uses—for treating headaches, arthritis and other forms of pain, insomnia, and as a poison—it was Arab traders who promoted and spread the plant. In around 330 BC it was introduced to Persia and India. By 400 AD opium had arrived in China.

From the Middle Ages onward, increased documentation indicates both the growing number of medicinal uses and benefits of the substance as well as a growing concern for its habit-forming tendencies. French naturalist and pharmacist Pierre Belon, writing in 1546, said of the popularity of the substance in the Ottoman Empire, "There is not a Turk who would not purchase opium with his last coin; he carries the drug on him in war and in peace. They eat opium because they

---

5. This text conflates terms in favor of the colloquial shorthand the "*opioid* epidemic," except where the technical specificities of the distinction, such as questions of production and sourcing (the Earth's soil versus a chemistry lab) are under examination.

think they will thus become more courageous and have less fear of the dangers of war."[6] A Portuguese doctor traveling in 1655 documented warnings about the drug's habit-forming nature from Indian, Malay, Chinese, Malabarian, Arab, Persian, and Turkish doctors. While early methods of intake involved imbibing opium, usually mixed with wine or honey to mask its bitterness, it is the Portuguese who are believed to have introduced the method of smoking opium in the 1500s, though some suggest Dutch traders introduced the practice after having been inspired by the Native American practice of tobacco smoking. The constricting atmosphere of the Inquisition and Reformation limited innovation involving opium in Europe, but with the dawning of the Renaissance, medical curiosity about the drug returned to public light and a slew of patent medicines containing opium began to emerge.

Two concoctions from opium took the name "laudanum." The first was in the form of pills containing crushed pearls. Their inventor, the sixteenth-century Swiss alchemist and healer Paracelsus, touted them as "stones of immortality." The other, an alcohol-based tincture, became widely popular in England and America in the 1800s as one of the most popular, and most dependency-inducing of the patent medicines of the time. This preparation is still available by prescription in the US and EU, though use is uncommon. Opium preparations, laudanum and paregoric, travelled with the pilgrims on the Mayflower, arriving in the Americas in 1620.[7]

MARKING THE OPIOID EPIDEMIC

Neither a natural disaster nor an anomaly, neither a grand conspiracy nor the work of a few bad actors, the opioid crisis was produced according to capital's logic and is one among countless articulations of capitalism's endemic pattern of producing plunder and pain for the sake of profit. The opioid crisis represents the integral devastation of life lived in capital's image and offers an opportunity to illuminate and question humankind's passive consent to structuring all of life in pursuit of abstracted and accumulating wealth above all other goals.

---

6.   Martin Booth, *Opium: A History* (New York: St. Martin's Griffin, 1999), 25.
7.   Th. Metzger, *The Birth of Heroin and the Demonization of the Dope Fiend* (Port Townsend, WA: Breakout Productions Inc., 1998).

Capitalism, a renovation on legacies of imperial violence, succeeds in surviving amidst its constantly produced crisis formations because it so pervasively supplants its own logics onto our collective ways of knowing and being human together. Born of compounding legacies of more obviously and visibly brutal regimes of domination and control for the sake of extraction, capitalism's staying power rests in its essential slippage, what I call in this work *the departure from the real*.

The opioid crisis, constructed from overlapping societal ills that have congealed into the present historical conjuncture, offers an opportunity to follow tethers that span the length of empire's global ambitions and allows us to look with curious new eyes on the conventions of the present world disorder. Through the kaleidoscope of histories that connect to the present crisis, we see the necessary coupling of pain and profit in the long history of market, commodity, and abstracted wealth-based social relations, and the stories that get told to partition people, communities, and consciousness in the service of ongoing domination.

Trying to make a life in academia required me to regurgitate death statistics on the crisis so much that I can barely manage the embodied cognitive and emotional labor required to include this data, but any book on the opioid epidemic must inform the unacquainted reader. Echoing my lost comrade David's remarks in the shadow of Our Lady of Victory that New England summer evening in 2015, I encourage you, dear reader, to take a moment before reading the next paragraph. I invite you to feel the energetic center of your living body, maybe just above or below your belly button. I invite you to breathe into this place while we name, and thus pay homage to, the lives lost.

Often in an unconscious attempt to remain resilient amidst the overwhelming preponderance of senseless violence and loss of life, we can confront accounts of violence and suffering as mere data to compute with our left brain before moving on for more content. Becoming ecosystemic requires us to feel and honor our feelings. Feel your own aliveness as you engage with the statistics I'm about to list here. I encourage you, as I am now, to be with the gnawing in your gut about the premature and preventable loss of life I'm about to catalogue; not because there's something special or moral about feeling it, but because feeling our grief and rage without being taken under in waves of powerlessness is a requisite for developing true resilience in these times. Do it because acknowledging our pain is essential for uncovering necessary and deeper truths out from the shadows of our individual and collective consciousness. Because reclaiming our hurt reconnects us to the web of life, and because refusing to be robotic computational devices is the real source of quantum intelligence.

Randy Martin remarked, "We can judge capital's reign not only by the riches and misery it produces, but also by its own promise to enrich the way we are together."[8] The Centers for Disease Control (CDC) reported 107,543 drug overdose deaths in 2023, a three percent decrease from 2022, marking only the second year of declining deaths since the introduction of OxyContin to the US healthcare landscape, which mainstreamed the prescribing of all kinds of opioids for non-terminal illness related pain. In 1995, the year of the drug's December FDA approval, there were 8,052 overdose deaths recorded by the CDC. The total number of prematurely lost American lives due to overdoses between 1999 and 2023 is 1.1 million. Of these premature deaths, 75 percent involved opioids and opiates.[9] From some vantages, American life in the last decade has been consumed by the opioid epidemic. It is a significant factor in the reversal of life expectancy numbers in the US. County morgues across the country are overburdened with the bodies of overdose victims.[10] A rash of coroner resignations began around 2013, with workers citing PTSD resulting from being inundated so suddenly in their daily work with prematurely dead people in the prime of life.[11] Municipalities all over the country cite skyrocketing rates of spending on first responder pay, jailing, and other associated costs. Families and communities struggle to remember a time before the issue consumed their attention and resources. A February 2024

8.   Randy Martin, *Financialization of Daily Life* (Philadelphia: Temple University Press, 2002), 7.

9.   Centers for Disease Control, "SUDORS Dashboard: Fatal Drug Overdose Data," CDC State Unintentional Drug Overdose Reporting System (SUDORS), February 26, 2024, https://www.cdc.gov/overdose-prevention/data-research/facts-stats/sudors-dashboard-fatal-overdose-data.html.

10.   Jordan Kisner, "Piled Bodies, Overflowing Morgues: Inside America's Autopsy Crisis," *New York Times*, February 25, 2020, sec. Magazine, https://www.nytimes.com/2020/02/25/magazine/piled-bodies-overflowing-morgues-inside-americas-autopsy-crisis.html.

11.   Raymond B. Flannery and Thomas Greenhalgh, "Coroners and PTSD: Treatment Implications," *Psychiatric Quarterly* 89, no. 4 (2018): 765–770.

study reported that 40 percent of American adults have lost someone to an overdose.[12]

Drug overdose is now the leading cause of death for Americans under fifty, with nearly double the fatalities of the next two highest causes of premature American death, car accidents and gunshots. A longstanding shortage in transplant organs has been remedied by the glut of prematurely dead people produced by the crisis.[13] Municipal water supplies and even shellfish off the coast of Seattle have been found to contain detectable amounts of opioids.[14]

The production and exacerbation of the crisis can be periodized in four marked waves. A glut of opioid prescribing occurred in the wake of Purdue Pharma and its cohort's aggressive and often covert marketing campaigns. The FDA approval for the drug came in late 1995. It is well documented that the trend in doctors prescribing opioids for prolonged use for chronic, non-terminal-cancer-related pain began earlier than the debut of OxyContin, the first drug approved for this purpose. The campaign (discussed more in Chapter 3) included sophisticated organizing to shape government policy and medical best-practices, intentional salesforce saturation in medical deserts flush with in-pain and out-of-work people with Medicare cards, and targeted marketing, lobbying, and sales pushes in states with lax or no prescription drug monitoring programs.[15]

The results produced a veritable free-flowing tap of the drugs from American doctors and pharmacies into patients' hands and home medicine cabinets. In 2011, about 131 million prescriptions for hydrocodone-containing medications, amounting to more than five billion pills, were written for about 47 million patients, according to CDC figures. In 2015 the number of legal and recorded prescriptions for opioid analgesics filled at American pharmacies was more than

12.   Alison Athey, Beau Kilmer, and Julie Cerel, "An Overlooked Emergency: More Than One in Eight US Adults Have Had Their Lives Disrupted by Drug Overdose Deaths," *American Journal of Public Health* 114, no. 3 (February 2024): 276–279.

13.   H. Boone and D. L. Gorden, "The Tragic Paradox of the 'Opioid Crisis' and Donors for Liver Transplantation: Increasing Organ Utilization in Recent Years," *HPB* 20 (September 1, 2018): https://www.hpbonline.org/article/S1365-182X(18)33811-5/fulltext.

14.   "Mussels off the Coast of Seattle Test Positive for Opioids," *CBS News*, May 24, 2018, https://www.cbsnews.com/news/mussels-test-positive-for-opioids-seattle-puget-sound/.

15.   Harriet Ryan, Lisa Girion, and Scott Glover, "'You Want a Description of Hell?' Oxy-Contin's 12-Hour Problem," *Los Angeles Times*, May 5, 2016, http://www.latimes.com/projects/OxyContin-part1/.

300 million, according to a 2016 market analyst by Mizuho Securities, a figure that led the then US Surgeon General Vivek Murthy to remark that enough prescriptions for opioids were written in that year for each American to have their own thirty-day supply.

The second phase (2010–2015) began when some states started clamping down on opioid overprescribing and opioid-dependent pain pill patients turned instead to heroin. A young woman in Portland who appears in a *New York Times* video report from 2013 titled, "In Maine, A Growing Heroin Menace," responds to the off-camera reporter's question as to why the sudden spike in heroin users in the state matter-of-factly: "Because there's no Oxys."[16] The timing of the report, along with the Maine legislature's tightening of restrictions on prescriptions for opioids, predictably coincided with a tripling of overdose deaths that year. The heroin being trafficked to Maine was extremely strong, even before fentanyl entered the picture, and extremely cheap. Increased demand encouraged a glut of supply, and for a while heroin was the cheapest street high available, and much cheaper than getting drunk on alcohol.[17] A national survey of new heroin users from 2014, which was regularly cited by the CDC and even former US President Obama, indicated that three out of four new heroin users in the 2003–2013 period reported first becoming dependent on prescription opioids, while other reports cite even higher figures.[18]

The third deadly wave of spiking death rates in the epidemic began in 2015 when the combined effect of further clampdowns on pill access collided, devastatingly, with the introduction of (mostly illicit, Chinese laboratory-produced) fentanyl into the supposed white-powder heroin supply chain. From 2016 to 2017 the rate of synthetic-opioid related death rose by 45.2 percent. The CDC also reported a "skyrocketing" rate of teenage overdose deaths in the 2014–2016 period, as illicit and extremely potent fentanyl and its analogs found their way into counterfeit pressed pills, many of which entered the US supply chain via Canada—an opioid trade route first established after the US reformulation of OxyContin encouraged the trafficking of the old, more

16.   Brent McDonald, "In Maine, a Growing Heroin Menace," *New York Times*, July 19, 2013, http://www.nytimes.com/video/us/100000002340382/a-deadly-dance.html.

17.   McDonald, "In Maine, a Growing Heroin Menace."

18.   Theodore J. Cicero et al., "The Changing Face of Heroin Use in the United States: A Retrospective Analysis of the Past 50 Years," *JAMA Psychiatry* 71, no. 7 (July 1, 2014): 821–826.

easily injectable formulation from Canadian pharmacies. Fentanyl first appeared clandestinely cut into heroin or was mixed with other cheap, white powdery substances and sold as heroin. However, by now sale and consumption of fentanyl happens overtly and on purpose. The potency of the drug produces its own demand, given how quickly tolerance builds to opioids in the human body.

After two decades of exponential growth in the rate of overdose deaths nationwide, numbers declined slightly for the first time in 2018. The decline can be attributed largely to the more widespread availability of naloxone, the overdose reversal drug, and the knowledge of, and habituation to, fentanyl-strength dope in the illicit, formerly, and formally "heroin" supply chain.

The COVID-19 pandemic marks the start of a fourth wave. Stress and isolation, along with the disruption of treatment and support services, provoked a new surge of deaths, with a 14 percent increase in deaths between 2020 and 2021. Additionally, a new trend of combining opioids with the veterinary tranquilizer xylazine, the combination of which is called "tranq" or "tranq dope" on the street, is producing a new emergency akin to the early fentanyl days. A July 2023 study concluded that the animal sedative was present in more than 90 percent of dope (injectable opioids, now largely presumed to be fentanyl-based) in Philadelphia.[19] With the multiplication of crises squeezing the topic out of the headlines, the opioid epidemic rages on with no resolution in sight. Ad hoc response measures at different scales of government belie a jumbled and piecemeal approach, with the most effective efforts being initiated by civilians and at the local level.

ADDICTION AND CAPITALISM

If we seek to understand the opioid epidemic, or addiction in general, including the current system's addictions to debt, oil, planetary plunder, and war-making, we're asking the same set of questions: why do humans act against their own self, or species, interest? Why do humans choose short-term gain that produces long-run pain? How

---

19. Ashley Schwartz-Lavares et al., "Community Groups, Medical Experts Work to Combat the Widespread 'Tranq' Drug Crisis," *ABC News*, https://abcnews.go.com/US/community-groups-medical-experts-work-combat-emerging-tranq/story?id=101716074.

did we come to inhabit a world that values this short-term orientation and produces pain-for-gain trade-offs?

In capital's image, life is thrown out of balance in pursuit of extraction, and humans consume commodities in a futile attempt to replace what has been lost, to recover from what has been severed, and to quell an inner knowledge that life ought to be something entirely otherwise. Humans turn to consumption-based coping mechanisms as a temporary salve for the aches induced by the present world disorder, which impoverishes our sense of reality and conscripts life's symphony of incommensurable and interrelated parts into a crass, reductive arithmetic.

The project to make capital's imperial violence rational, reasonable, sensible, and orderly relies on flattening the dimensions of our spatial and temporal ways of knowing. Capitalism's staying power is that it has grafted its logic onto not only how we live but how we think about life. While it, like all human systems and inventions, is of course animated by human actors, its real grip on the collective is that it subsumes human sensibilities to its impersonal rationale. Moishe Postone described it as "the domination of people by abstract social structures that people themselves constitute."[20] More recently, David Harvey has called it "the madness of economic reason."[21]

The ongoing present (dis)order of things rests on partition and domination: the departure from the real, forced forgetting, and the persistence of a violent past in the present. Partition and domination, dualism, structures everything in the dead but dominant paradigm, from our individual sense of self-and-other, self-in-context, and self itself. Partition produced the exile and degradation of our bodies' intelligence apart from our minds and thwarts our understanding of humans as a part of Earth's ecosystemic functions. In rendering the embedded and essential violence that produced and prolongs capitalism as invisible, normal, natural or inevitable, the capitalist system produces human beings with a severed consciousness, forced to bear the cognitive, embodied, and social weight of the system's disowned contradictions.

---

20. Moishe Postone, *Time, Labor, and Social Domination* (Cambridge and New York: Cambridge University Press, 1996), 30.
21. David Harvey, *Marx, Capital, and the Madness of Economic Reason* (New York: Oxford University Press, 2017).

MAPPING THE WAY HOME

As John Berger teaches us, "A large part of seeing is about habit and convention."[22] Before we can name the locus of harm done in the opioid crisis, we must acknowledge the backdrop, the erasures and blinders and partitions in our own consciousness that renders the pursuit of profit and plunder normalized and naturalized.

Capitalism is a sickness that pursues abstract and compounding wealth as an organizing principle for all of life. The project to make capital's imperial violence rational, reasonable, sensible, and orderly required colonizing not only our Earth but our minds, our beliefs, our consciousness. All people, including the ancestors of people who became white, had to be stripped of their indigeneity. Our very sense of self, life, purpose, and meaning had to be shredded for the virus of compound growth to take hold and spread. Securing its ongoing operation requires that this state of erasure and displacement must continually be maintained.

In the capitalist world disorder, human beings live in exile, lost without a map. Robbed of a language and framework for taking sufficient account of the depth and dimensions of an inherently relational, ecosystemic order to life, we can't locate ourselves sufficiently in the present. This geographical, historical, relational reckoning, a type of re-homing, is an essential component to becoming agents of revolutionary change. We are tasked with reconstructing the spacetime of the world, to make new maps, new collective meaning. We must scout for common ground.

22. John Berger, *Ways of Seeing* (New York: Penguin, 1972).

CHAPTER 2

TEACHING ECONOMICS AT THE END OF THE PARADIGM

One of the key themes in microeconomics is the validity of Adam Smith's insight: individuals pursuing their own interests often do promote the interests of society as a whole.

—Paul Krugman and Robin Wells, *Microeconomics* (2017)

We don't suffer from being individuals, we suffer from trying to be that. . . . Since the individual entity exists, fictitiously, only from the outside, 'being an individual' requires remaining outside oneself, strangers to ourselves, forgoing any contact with oneself as well as with the world and others.

—The Invisible Committee, *Now* (2017)

In the spring of 2019, at the end of my one-year position as Visiting Assistant Professor in Macroeconomics at the University of Southern Maine, I pared down my belongings for a transatlantic move. Picking up my Intermediate Microeconomics problem set binder—that I'd inexplicably kept for nearly twenty years—I flipped through hundreds of pages of plotted logarithmic functions determining maximum utils. I felt a pang of grief, reflecting on the lost life force and tuition money. Utils represent discrete units of abstract "utility," or consumer satisfaction, which the discipline conflates with happiness and well-being. "This is how busy microeconomics keeps you, hoping you don't stop to think about the underlying fucking premise!" I said to my friend while tossing it in the discard pile. Later I carried it to the dumpster my then-home shared with the homeless shelter next door. Before heaving it in, I luckily noticed two people living in a tent at the bottom of the dumpster. I offered a startled greeting, left the bag, and turned back toward my house. In my headphones, Kendrick Lamar rapped, "Ain't a profit big enough to feed you."[1]

"How the fuck is a 4-4 a VAP?" my protective friend Rachel dared ask me, referring to the fact that the job contract required teaching four courses per semester, whereas my tenured colleagues mostly taught two or at most three. Accepting the job contract represented an instance of what economists might call "irrational exuberance" and what Lauren Berlant would have sniffed out as "cruel optimism."

Nine years into my PhD, having leveraged my personal debt worthiness beyond acceptable standards even to the federal government, and coming from a family which, in my mother's words, *don't got two dimes to rub together*, I had run out of conceivable ways to pay for my staying alive while writing the dissertation. So, in a cognitive rupture from reality, I decided I could do it all—teach four courses a semester, finish my dissertation, apply for jobs, and sure, even write a journal article or two. In my father's terms, it was *a Hail Mary pass with seconds on the clock*, but with me needing to both throw and catch the ball. The choice set of the post-Reagan, blue-collar American working class: go big or go homeless.

In the fall, I teach three sections of Macroeconomics 101 and one Money and Banking course. My students are veterans who have survived several deployments to Iraq and Afghanistan for a chance at the GI Bill as well as immigrants and refugees who have survived and fled from those same and other wars. My students leave lecture to take calls from insurance companies about denial of coverage for their spouse's cancer treatment. My students are responsible for younger siblings in the wake of a parent's sudden deportation. My students are curious about, possibly participants in, or rightly terrified of recently emboldened far-right campus activity. My students are self-medicating anxiety and depression. My students have court dates, or work two hours shy of benefits-qualifying full-time at near-minimum wage. My students have emergency psychiatric hospital admissions. My students come to office hours to ask *me* for advice about how to have a successful future. They are cynical, but curious and open, trying

---

1.   Kendrick Lamar, "Alright," 2015, Track 7 on *To Pimp a Butterfly*, Aftermath Entertainment, LP.

to navigate life in this world without sufficient knowledge or understanding to comprehend the present or to locate themselves in it. My
students are lost without a map.

FORCED FORGETTING

Forced forgetting is a project of erasure and the essence and extent
of the hermeneutic violence baked into the present paradigm. I elaborate on the concept of hermeneutic violence in Chapter 5. In short
it is the violence of erasure of knowledge and context that produces a
false sense of reality and that hobbles the capacity to make meaning
or meaningful change. Forced forgetting is essential to the creation of
knowledge systems based in abstractions and social (dis)orders based
on quantification.

The production of abstract space is a necessary precursor to a
social disorder predicated on abstract wealth. It makes uniformity,
order, out of the beautiful mess of life lived in context, in place, on
a living Earth. In his 1973 book *How Europe Underdeveloped Africa*,
Walter Rodney writes about the differences between Indigenous and
colonial education. The colonial regime "civilized" children by teaching them civilized-people things, like how to identify and spell the
names of European flowers. Rodney says that Indigenous education,
by contrast, was divorced neither from spirit nor intellect. Children
would learn, in ways that were age appropriate and useful, things like
which flora surround them and keep them alive. Students in economics classes, seeking to learn something useful, are often educated out
of recognizing what matters for survival.

In addition to the requisite content, I do what a good geographer
does—I teach my students to read the landscape, to think spatially
about economic processes. Economic ontology abstracts space and
time into linear two-variable two-axis models, which detach the theory
from applicability and relevance. The discipline's foundations rest on
axioms and regurgitations reminiscent of what psychiatrist Robert Jay
Lifton named "thought-terminating cliches."[2] Its linguistic devices and

---

2.   Robert Jay Lifton, *Thought Reform and the Psychology of Totalism: A Study of "Brainwashing"*
in China (Chapel Hill: University of North Carolina Press, 1989).

signifiers quiet cognitive dissonance over too simplistic or otherwise unsatisfactory explanations. When talking about economic restructuring, it is common to hear an economist sound like a personal trainer—No Pain, No Gain.[3] Devoid of spatiality, the models neglect to inquire: whose pain is whose gain? The dominant paradigm insists that a rising tide lifts all boats and offers moralistic or pseudoscientific explanations for all the wrecked vessels in our midst. With allusions to Darwin and other instantiations of cutthroat "human nature," actors deploying economic logic to justify pain-for-gain tradeoffs shrug off these questions as simply the cold facts—life is about winners and losers in a zero-sum game.

The discipline of economics constructs a nearly impenetrable smokescreen by presenting the supposed science as both simple and sophisticated. It exemplifies what Neil Smith articulates as the "essential dualism" of nature that shaped Western scientific thought—that nature, somehow at once, exists outside of and separate from humanity, yet that human history can be explained by a reductive concept of human nature and its evolution.[4] "Economics is a young science," said Harvard economist and author of a popular undergraduate economic textbook, Greg Mankiw in a 2010 essay.[5] Mankiw goes on to list what he claims are "general laws," that which "we economists are confident is true," including supply and demand and the theory of comparative advantage. Einstein, in a 1949 essay, by contrast, remarked that elevating the discipline of economics to a "science" was not reasonable, saying that the discovery of general laws in the field couldn't be observed in the abstract, as economic phenomena is never abstract, and that in the "'so-called civilized' period of human history," present conditions and economic phenomena cannot be considered outside of the context of "conquest."[6] The reductive quantifications the discipline uses

3. Graciela Kaminsky and Sergio L. Schmukler, "Short-Run Pain, Long-Run Gain: The Effects of Financial Liberalization," SSRN Scholarly Paper (Rochester, NY: Social Science Research Network, June 1, 2003), https://papers.ssrn.com/abstract=418289.

4. Neil Smith, *Uneven Development: Nature, Capital, and the Production of Space* (Athens: University of Georgia Press, 2008).

5. N. Gregory Mankiw, "Crisis Economics" (Summer 2010), *National Affairs* 59 (Spring 2024), https://www.nationalaffairs.com/publications/detail/crisis-economics.

6. Albert Einstein, "Why Socialism?," *Monthly Review* 1, no. 1 (May 1949).

to model social phenomena evokes Henri Lefebvre's assertion that abstract space is "a product of violence and war."[7]

In public discourse, economists alternately present economic logic as a 'no brainer' and as 'rocket science.' Economics and finance employ astoundingly complex, quantum equations to model, explain, and predict economic events predicated on foundational concepts that are themselves two-dimensional. When state-finance nexus titans petitioned Warren Buffet for a massive investment in the mortgage sector to save the global economy in 2008, Buffet swiftly declined. "I looked at one offering of mortgage-backed securities. I would've had to read over 300,000 pages [of data] to analyze that mortgage."[8] As physicist and former Goldman Sachs quantitative analyst Emanuel Derman put it, "Economists love formal mathematics much more than physicists do. Many economic journals encourage—or even demand—a faux-rigorous style with multitudes of axioms and lemmas in numbers that tend to be inversely proportional to their efficacy in the real world."[9]

All wealth, whether mediated through a money mechanism or other measure, comes from the Earth and the applied human labor that turns nature's bounty into socially useful abundance. This is the Labor Theory of Value (LTV), articulated by David Ricardo in *Principles of Political Economy and Taxation* (1817), and taken up by the philosophers who became the first political economists and the intellectual founding fathers of the discipline of economics. Nearly all the classical political economists between Ricardo and Marx's times accepted the LTV until the formidable logical and moral conundrums within it became apparent. If living labor was the source of value, how did one explain why the vast majority of the laborers who produce said value lived in squalor? Whether industrial workers in urban slums or the remaining agricultural workers living in degraded circumstances in the countryside, the intellectual handmaidens of the burgeoning school of classical economic thought could neither deny this fact nor explain it in accordance with the LTV. The question was taken up by a

7.   Henri Lefebvre, *The Production of Space*, trans. Donald Nicholson-Smith (Malden: Wiley-Blackwell, 1992), 285.
8.   *PANIC! The Untold Story of the 2008 Financial Crisis*, directed by John Maggio (2018; Washington, DC and New York: HBO Documentary, Vice News and Ark Media), HBO.
9.   Emanuel Derman, "Beware of Economists Bearing Greek Symbols," *Harvard Business Review*, October 1, 2005, https://hbr.org/2005/10/beware-of-economists-bearing-greek-symbols.

group who came to be known as the Ricardian Socialists, but was otherwise sidelined in the mainstream, where the discussion of the moral problem, and the LTV itself, were effectively dropped.

Intellectual tradition in the time of Ricardo placed a great deal of emphasis on abstract thought. This penchant for abstraction still undergirds the discipline of economics today. Doing away with questions of value, the discipline of economics as it congealed, focused its theory and model-making practically exclusively on the power of the price mechanism to orchestrate a seemingly perfect union of supply and demand.[10] Two-axis, price-quantity modeling hereafter became a central focus of theoretical and intellectual pursuit within economics. The fetishization of the price mechanism, and the two-axis supply and demand modeling that retains centrality in the discipline as taught in universities, draws frustration and ire from students seeking to understand how the economy actually functions.[11]

In the Money and Banking course, we discuss the myth of barter, the "thought experiment" reproduced in nearly every account of the nature of money in nearly every introductory economics textbook. We discuss the idea that money developed because trading cheese for chickens was cumbersome and imprecise. The premise suggests that economics has always existed or has evolved naturally to a quantified tit-for-tat exchange of abstracted equal units of value, when in fact, in the words of Cambridge anthropologist Caroline Humphrey, "All available ethnography suggests that there never has been such a thing."[12]

We discuss the implications of the historical and anthropological studies of money that demonstrate that barter only seems to have existed in circumstances where people accustomed to money-based exchange don't have money, such as in prisons. In contrast to the thought experiment of barter, historical accounts suggest that compulsory participation in money and market-based exchange emerges out of lordly ambitions to conquer more *tierra firma*, namely the practical matter of provisioning armies on the march.

10.   Robert L. Heilbroner, *The Worldly Philosophers: The Lives, Times and Ideas of the Great Economic Thinkers* (New York: Touchstone, 1999), 135.

11.   "Harvard Students to Walk Out on Mankiw," *Nation*, November 1, 2011, https://www.thenation.com/article/archive/harvard-students-walk-out-mankiw/.

12.   Caroline Humphrey, "Barter and Economic Disintegration," *Man* 20, no. 1 (1985): 48–72.

I ask my students what they think of the implications. A student who almost never speaks looks up, "It's like the fourth wall drops."

BEYOND THE FOURTH WALL

The "free market," "the invisible hand," and "free trade," among other axioms, are thought-terminating cliches that serve as antidotes to the ontological partitions embedded in economics. In collapsing critical dimensions of space and time the discipline papers over our capacity for seeing and knowing self, other, the collective, and "the economy." By adding depth and dimension, we see the tethers that connect the imperialist past to the present. The general law of comparative advantage put forth by Ricardo in 1817, demonstrates the win-win of specialization and trade cooperation. The example of English wool for Portuguese wine is still touted as catechism by prominent contemporary economists and used in current debates in support of (race to the bottom) free trade agreements. Columbia University economist Ronald Findlay called Ricardo's theory of comparative advantage "the deepest and most beautiful result in all of economics."[13] Meanwhile in the real world, both countries at the time of Ricardo's writing were nearly two hundred years into the triangular slave trade.

Anthropologist Sidney Mintz says of the historical fact of triangular trade:

> The important feature of these triangles is that human cages figured vitally in their operation. It was not just that sugar, rum, and molasses that were not being traded directly for European finished goods; in both transatlantic triangles the only "false commodity"—yet absolutely essential to the system—was human beings. Slaves were a "false commodity" because a human being is not an object, even when treated as one. In this instance, millions of human beings were treated as commodities. To obtain them, products were shipped to Africa; by their labor power, wealth was created in the Americas. The wealth they created mostly returned to Britain; the products they made were consumed in Britain; and the products made by Brit-

---

13. Roger Lowenstein, "TPP and Free Trade: Why Congress Should Listen to the World's Richest Economist," *Fortune*, June 22, 2015, http://fortune.com/2015/06/22/top-fast-track-david-ricardo/.

ons—cloth, tools, torture instruments—were consumed by slaves who were themselves consumed in the creation of wealth.[14]

As with most classical economic models, the appeal of comparative advantage is in its simplicity. It speaks to a certain common sense, an intuitive, smarter-not-harder collective ethos. The discipline of economics still wears the guise of being something like scientific. Ricardo's theory of comparative advantage posits an even geopolitical terrain where cooperation and mutual agreements benefit everyone, and no negotiating ever happened from either end of the barrel of a gun. Paul Krugman, defending contemporary free trade agreements against opposed "intellectuals who are interested in economic issues" said that they "refuse to sit still for the ten minutes or so it takes to explain Ricardo."[15]

A prime example of an economic axiom is *assume perfect information*—the presumption that all parties to economic transactions know everything needed to make an optimal decision. Yet uneven information, power, and persuasion are central to the acquisition of profit. *Assume perfect information* also fails the contemporary relevance test considering the recent revelations of the Paradise, Panama, and Pandora Papers: the ubiquity of not only tax dodging but the prevalence of completely anonymous, yet politically active, post-national capital is a direct contradiction to the somehow still-uttered notion that "free markets" promote democracy. Headlines are rife with evidence of the melding of licit and illicit capital,[16] the degree to which banks depend on criminal cartel money to remain solvent,[17] international actors stirring political chaos and tipping the scales in favor of

---

14.   Sidney Wilfred Mintz, *Sweetness and Power: The Place of Sugar in Modern History* (New York: Penguin Books, 1986), 43.

15.   Paul Krugman, "Ricardo's Difficult Idea: Why Intellectuals Don't Understand Comparative Advantage," in Gary Cook (ed.), *The Economics and Politics of International Trade* (London: Routledge, 1998).

16.   Louise Story and Stephanie Saul, "Stream of Foreign Wealth Flows to Elite New York Real Estate," *New York Times*, February 7, 2015, sec. New York, https://www.nytimes.com/2015/02/08/nyregion/stream-of-foreign-wealth-flows-to-time-warner-condos.html.

17.   Spencer Woodman, "HSBC Moved Vast Sums of Dirty Money after Paying Record Laundering Fine – ICIJ," September 21, 2020, https://www.icij.org/investigations/fincen-files/hsbc-moved-vast-sums-of-dirty-money-after-paying-record-laundering-fine/; Rajeev Syal, "Drug Money Saved Banks in Global Crisis, Claims UN Advisor," *Observer*, December 13, 2009, sec. World News, https://www.theguardian.com/global/2009/dec/13/drug-money-banks-saved-un-cfief-claims.

far-right candidates,[18] and the fact that vested interests will murder to protect imperfect information.[19] Economics tells us to assume perfect information in a social order rife with obstruction and intentional disinformation.

Mankiw says the "business cycle," the term economists use for the fact of economic downturns and crises, is the least well understood of all of the so-called general laws of economics. The underspecified theory of the business cycle presents crises as an act of God, naturalizing and mystifying capitalism's crisis-prone nature. Two-dimensional, boom-bust models flatten out the geography of uneven development and ignore one of Marx's crucial insights about the spatial dimensions of capitalist growth and its resulting circulation problems. In theorizing the business cycle, economists ignore the fact that compound growth is a territorial project and that compound growth on a finite planet damns us all.

In the immediate wake of the 2008–2009 crisis, economic analysts began debating the efficacy of the business cycle models used in the state-finance response effort. Yet, former Treasury Secretary Henry Paulson admits that his strategy was never about macro-fundamentals. Regarding the congressional approval process, a hostile takeover, Paulson said, "I looked at those hearings as largely theater," intending to secure a blank check, or "unspecified authority," to calm global markets. "If you've got a squirt gun in your pocket, you may have to take it out. If you've got a bazooka, and people know you've got it, you may not have to take it out."[20]

Highly technical macroeconomic modeling seemed secondary to simple arithmetic as proponents of the free market joined efforts to organize its rescue in a series of actions that looked a lot like the dreaded p-word, "planning." In the days after the collapse of Lehman Brothers, a secret meeting was convened at the White House with what journalist Andrew Sorkin called "the five families" of Wall Street,

---

18. "Cambridge Analytica: The Data Firm's Global Influence," *BBC News*, March 22, 2018, sec. World, https://www.bbc.com/news/world-43476762.

19. Juliette Garside, "Malta Car Bomb Kills Panama Papers Journalist," *Guardian*, October 16, 2017, sec. World news, https://www.theguardian.com/world/2017/oct/16/malta-car-bomb-kills-panama-papers-journalist.

20. *PANIC!*

including Jamie Dimon and Lloyd Blankfein. Sorkin remarked, "[T] hey were effectively being given an assignment. Hank and Tim are the schoolteachers telling the children, you're gonna be broken up into groups to come up with a deal to ring-fence these [toxic] assets."[21]

Aspatial, ahistorical economic ontology theorizes an overtly reductive concept of "the state" and "the market" as diametrically opposing forces, occluding the historical and present-day realities of state-market entwinement. In 2008, when Paulson asked former Federal Reserve Chairman Alan Greenspan for suggestions for stabilizing the economy, he offered a simple supply-and-demand inspired strategy—"buy and burn" vacant homes.[22] Later telling reporters that he understood the policy was "not viable politically," he maintained that, in theory, it was the best strategy.[23] Ignoring the premise of the general law of supply and demand, and of the fundamentalist orthodoxy of the market's self-regulating capacity, Greenspan and Paulson's interventions reveal another blatant contradiction: sometimes the invisible hand works for the state and wields a bazooka, or kerosene and a match.

The theory of the business cycle, not mentioning people or distribution, ignores the implicit deterioration of life circumstances of the expropriated class. In discussion and essays, many of my students disclose their personal connections to the financial crisis—foreclosure, decimated family savings, bankruptcy, and divorce. Several attribute their motivation for enlisting in the military to their family's financial ruin. Economists also like to refer to economic crises as a "correction," like an unpleasant trip to the chiropractor. No pain, no gain.

BESPOKE ACCUMULATION AND HUMANITARIAN CRISIS

In October, with my first paycheck, I buy a used car from an acquaintance, a friend of many friends in a small community. She and her boyfriend tend bar part-time and have just bought a house thanks

---

21.   *PANIC!* The "Hank and Tim" referred to here are Hank Paulson and Tim Geithner, respectively US Treasury secretary and president of the New York Fed during the "great financial crisis of 2008."

22.   Andrew Ross Sorkin, *Too Big to Fail: The Inside Story of How Wall Street and Washington Fought to Save the Financial System—and Themselves* (London: Penguin Books, 2010).

23.   Jennifer Taub, *Other People's Houses* (New Haven: Yale University Press, 2014).

to the generosity of her wealthy parents. I am operating under an assumption of trust, what James Scott might call a "moral economy."[24] I take for granted that the price being offered is fair, that the condition and history of the car is truthfully disclosed. I assume this because I assume the seller is acting as a member of my community and not as an individuated business unit, a "rational economic actor."

I make my decision hastily. Among its other limitations, rational choice theory doesn't consider the neuropsychology of extreme stress. In a human brain experiencing survival fear, the amygdala decides, bypassing higher-order cognition. I beam her nearly all the money I've got to my name. Bad *Homo economicus*.

In November, the car breaks down and a few days later I learn it isn't worth the cost of fixing. In the *Grundrisse*, Marx remarks that under capitalism, money becomes the community only to destroy the community.[25] The Invisible Committee echo this observation, saying economics wages its war on the plane of our bonds to one another.[26] I lost the game of survival of the fittest again and I'm back on the bus. I am the only person on the bus who is not a homeless person, either trying to get somewhere or trying to get some sleep. I am the last off the bus at the last stop. The driver has a notably kind rapport with everyone who has gotten off the bus before me. He tells me his kindness comes from his own experience having been homeless for four years prior to securing the bus driving job less than a year ago.

"Thank god for this job," he says. "Thank god for kind people. I try to be a kind person because I know the difference it makes to someone in difficult circumstances."

I get off the bus at the coastline, where I once saw a mysterious unmarked vessel that turned out to be a Google data barge, slurping up free coolant from the fastest warming body of water in the world and dumping it back hot.[27] The disappearance of cod isn't the only survival threat plaguing fisherman here; the increased presence of

---

24. James C. Scott, *The Moral Economy of the Peasant: Rebellion and Subsistence in Southeast Asia* (New Haven: Yale University Press, 1977).
25. Karl Marx, *Grundrisse: Foundations of the Critique of Political Economy*, trans. Martin Nicolaus (New York: Penguin Classics, 1993), 224.
26. The Invisible Committee, *Now*, trans. Robert Hurley (South Pasadena: Semiotext(e), 2017).
27. Rory Carroll, "Google's Worst-Kept Secret: Floating Data Centers off US Coasts," *The Guardian*, October 30, 2013, http://www.theguardian.com/technology/2013/oct/30/google-secret-floating-data-centers-california-maine.

mega-yachts portends to crowd out dock space on the working water-front.[28] A new luxury condo a few blocks from home has just released marketing material that reminds me of the 2015 horror film *High-Rise*. Detailing a "day in the life" of a resident, the text reads: "Professional property management allows you to do the things you love. Lock your door and leave for the weekend or the month. Someone else will shovel the walk and remove the trash . . . [and] your latest Amazon order is safely stored." A friend jokes that the "typical day" in our recently named Restaurant City of the Year suggests a habitual daily intake of approximately 8,000 calories. Swing by an Instagram-friendly bakery newly opened by millennials migrating from Brooklyn for some buttery scones and pecan pie. Enjoy a "Roasted Acorn Squash Panini" and a poutine for lunch. Knock off early from your remote, laptop job and kick back with a couple of cold ones "brewed just five blocks away." "Yes, life really is this good.... Your new home is everything you hoped it would be. And more."[29] *Ever wanted something more? Join us at the High Rise.*

A friend gives me a ride. She is a grant administrator for a federal program targeting homeless veterans. She tells me the encampment she visited that day, where residents have chickens and a small vegetable garden, will be destroyed by police tomorrow; she spent her day strategizing with people who reside there about where they will go. I tell her what I've recently been piecing together about the city's debt burden, their latest Standard & Poor's rating report, how homelessness contradicts the unelected city manager's priority of ever-rising property values, the municipality's single asset, *tierra firma*, which secures its projected solvency and creditworthiness. My friend is furiously puffing on a vape pen while we drive, talking about her urgent need for a career change. We make an awful joke about homeless services being the only gig in town offering a 401k. She accelerates and brakes too quickly and expresses exasperation with fellow drivers. Catching herself, she laughs, embarrassed, "Don't mind me! Just another American *living on the edge!*"

---

28. Andrew J. Pershing et al., "Slow Adaptation in the Face of Rapid Warming Leads to Collapse of the Gulf of Maine Cod Fishery," *Science* 350, no. 6262 (November 13, 2015): 809–812.
29. NewHeight Group, "A day in the life of a Luminato resident," *Luminato*, August 10, 2016, https://luminatocondos.com/day-life-luminato-resident/.

Heading home in a taxi, I check a job posting on my phone and notice the university homepage dons a bold banner directed at current students: "Are you in crisis?" My taxi driver is a fifty-something woman suffering from chronic backpain. She has grappled with opioid addiction and has neither the credit score nor the cashflow to secure a nice enough car to drive for Uber. The scene of masses of homeless people obstructing my street is always a conversation starter.[30] We talk about how working-class people have been thrown away in the US, and how she was recently forced to move to a rundown factory town when her lifelong home was leveled and replaced by luxury condos for "people from away." "I want these fuckin' people to leave and give us our fuckin' town back," she says. A bumper sticker on a passing pickup truck, rigged for cement work, reads: "I'd be a liberal but I'm too busy working."

Early in the spring semester, I try to buy a burrito, and my card is declined. This is how I learn my bank account has been surprise-garnished by a debt shark. The term describes firms who buy defaulted, written-down debt on secondary markets and pursue collection often beyond the full extent of the law. I understand the mechanisms involved; the debt was acquired obtaining a Master of International Trade and Investment Policy. A friend with an architecture degree from a well-regarded school tends bar at the kind of place that's all white-tile, mounted deer heads, and sprigs of baby's breath on the tables (I think of Neil Smith's quip that gentrification in smaller towns reproduces the rural as the rustic). He buys me a drink on his shift, and I sit slurping in shock, laughing instead of crying about the contradictions I embody. Visiting Assistant Professor in Macroeconomics, without—my mother again—*a pot to piss in.* His coworker, also a university graduate, overhears our conversation and interjects, "But economics is kinda fake though, right?"

---

30. Randy Billings, "Bayside at Rock Bottom: Portland Neighborhood Is under Siege," *Press Herald*, May 6, 2018, https://www.pressherald.com/2018/05/06/bayside-at-rock-bottom-a-neighborhood-under-siege/.

CONSCIOUSNESS AND REVOLUTION

Just another human, species, planet, *living on the edge*. But the edge of what? Economics produces cognitive dislocation from the embodied, grounded present. It forecloses our individual and collective consciousness—the literal and perceptual ground we stand on and our tools for meaning-making. Understanding the dynamics of the present-in-context is a precursor to one or a collective's sense of reality and purpose. Orientation to the here and now is an essential component of imagining ourselves as agents of change in a viable future.

A paradigm shift is a revolution in thought, occurring when the old framework does not represent what we know to be true and does not allow us to ask, let alone answer, the right questions. As David Harvey put it in 1972, addressing the urgency for a post-quantitative turn in geography, "[T]here is a clear disparity between the sophisticated theoretical and methodological framework which we are using and our ability to say anything really meaningful about events as they unfold around us."[31] The discipline of economics, with its cognitive abstractions from space and time does not meet the standard of intellectual rigor required to produce new theory for conceiving new ways of being, making, and doing together, toward a livable, peaceable future. Situating ourselves in place is essential for understanding the economy and for seeing capitalism, so deft at hiding behind cliches and supposedly natural laws. A collective consciousness rooted in relational spacetime is necessary for producing economic policy that remembers, acknowledges, and reveres what it is to be human together on a living Earth. Historian and friend Sónia Vaz Borges puts it more sharply: "consciousness is the coming into awareness that you are colonized."[32] Beyond and distinct from ideology, epistemology and ontology, revolutions in consciousness entail the process of locating ourselves in a historical present with untold possible futures, to be determined by our individual and collective actions in the situated now.

---

31. David Harvey, "Revolutionary and Counter Revolutionary Theory in Geography," *Antipode* 17, no. 2–3 (1985): 24–27.
32. Sónia Vaz Borges, "Militant Education, Liberation Struggle, Consciousness," presentation in Migrations and Mobilizations: Revolutionary Internationalism Today, public event at the Center for Place, Culture and Politics, CUNY Graduate Center, April 12–13, 2017.

In the parking lot across the street from the homeless teen drop-in resource center, where disproportionally poor, traumatized, queer, and neurodivergent young people wash their laundry, dry their feet, and have a snack, an artist has installed a simple, white, three-by-four-feet wooden sign with black stick-on lettering: "You are here. You are reading this sign. You have made a choice."

CHAPTER 3

FINDING A FIX

I'm from the murder capital, where we murder for capital.

—Jay-Z, "Lucifer" (2003)[1]

Capitalism taps our veins, needs our flesh. The production of the opioid epidemic is an example of the extent to which the neoliberal turn
allowed for wholesale state capture by the capitalist class. Colluding as
a class to sell their dependency-inducing product, the Sacklers, among
other white-market drug dealers, bought institutional influence
through overt and covert channels in order not just to gain approval
to sell their product, but to change the very knowledge base of society. In a grand *golpe* of the collective conscious, advertising, covert
cash dressed as "advocacy," and slogans masquerading as advances in
medical science collided to change 10,000 years of collective common
sense about the safety of long-term opioid use. The case illustrates the
extent to which neoliberal global economic restructuring ushered in a
new phase in capital's empire. Segments of the American blue-collar
working class who had been the recipients of a degree of privilege
under the terms of racial and classed order since the so-called Progressive Era lost their standing, as a new phase of intensified extraction
and exploitation at a world scale no longer needed their labor or
their buy-in. The production of the opioid epidemic illustrates how
the shifting global order ruptured the ground under the feet of the
working class in formerly core, formally democratic parts of the world.

---

1.   Jay-Z, "Lucifer" (produced by Kanye West), track 12 on *The Black Album*, Roc-A-Fella
and Def Jam Records, 2003, CD.

Imperialist plunder—debt, extraction, prison, and pain—laid waste to life in place, destroying or outmaneuvering supposedly democratic checks and balances against the powers of the powerful to murder, seize, and destroy in the name of accumulation.

Capital's ambition is to become the state. Its stately ambitions revolve around its existential need to dominate people and the living Earth. The reasons for this are clear from a geographical perspective on the mechanics of capitalist accumulation. Critiques of capitalism in popular consciousness in the so-called Western world often over-emphasize the role of exploitation from waged labor relative to other tactics of capitalist growth. This feature, paying workers less than the value of the fruits of their labor, is called *surplus value extraction* and is the terrain of struggle for organized labor.

Another front of accumulation comes from extraction. Extraction takes place as mining from the Earth's veins, but also, crucially, from humans and other life forms' lifeforce. This, what David Harvey calls *accumulation by dispossession*, is an essential feature of the system. Recognition of it allows us to see the tethers connecting the supposedly "just" and "rational" system to its brutal, imperialist essence. A core feature of capitalism's quest for growth is that it turns human beings, all of life, and the Earth herself, into conduits for its valorization. Overlooking these essential features of capitalism limits our capacity to recognize one another as comrades in the same struggle, at this point in its global endgame, as a species.

Capital survives by tapping humans and our Earth mother's veins, by any means necessary—whether we're talking about Big Pharma or Big Oil, the Sinaloa Cartel or the Sackler Clan. The principal twinned impulses of extraction and dependency comprise the existential quest to resolve, always only temporarily, capital's inherent internal crisis. This need to possess a secure base, the Earth, our bodies, as conduits through which capital can flow, grow, and be realized as value, is essential to all the world's seemingly different contemporary crises. It is the thread connecting all our struggles.

To quote a track from one of the most personally influential albums of my teenage years: "Capitalism is indeed organized crime, and we are all the victims."[2] Because the system's logic debases every-thing but the central concern of the short-term, high-yield growth of capital, awareness of the catastrophic consequences in the future holds no power as an argument to change course in the present. Cli-mate collapse tomorrow has nothing on the imperative to get new oil and gas contracts signed today. Capital is running on fumes. The mer-ry-go-round of boom-bust-kaboom is reaching another full cycle in its revolution. It is not the actual oil that gives the system liquidity today. It is the paperwork—securities, contracts on the construction and futures on the predicted stream of revenues, that provides security to the financial system. The banking system, nation states and their currency regimes, must demonstrate the capacity to turn the Earth and its life forms into money in the bank. This is what reassures the markets. This is the crux of the present moment's heightened frenzy of extraction, from the North Sea to the Congo.

WORLD WAR FAST AND SLOW

The opioid epidemic is a byproduct of the post-1971 neoliberal *coup d'etat* of the global capitalist class.[3] In a renovation of earlier, more explicitly violent modes of imperial capture and conquest, the neolib-eral coup created an intensified regime of accumulation typified by an expansion and proliferation of financialized and extractivist tac-tics. Rentiership, debt arrangements, natural-resource capture, and other kinds of *golpe growth* strategies rose markedly in the neoliberal period.[4] When we follow the thread through the occluded history of how both capitalism and its knowledge regime, chiefly the discipline of economics, came to be, we see the truth hiding offstage. Capital-ism is less about 'value added' and more about asset stripping. *Golpe growth* allows us to see that we inhabit, are being done in by, an eco-nomic system where profit is generated by mining life-force itself. It happens at a multiplication of scales, from our Earth Mother herself

---

2.   Refused, "The Refused Party Program," track 7 on *The Shape of Punk to Come*, Burning Heart, 1998, CD.
3.   David Harvey, "Neoliberalism as Creative Destruction," *The Annals of the American Academy of Political and Social Science* 610 (2007): 22–44.
4.   David Harvey, "The 'New' Imperialism: Accumulation by Dispossession," *Socialist Register* 40 (2004), https://socialistregister.com/index.php/srv/article/view/5811.

and her life forms, including animals and human beings. Neoliberal economic restructuring intensified both the inherent violence of capitalism along with the system's embedded cognitive, spatial, and perceptual slippages.

The secret hidden in plain sight in the history of the so-called modern world reads as follows: phases of stagnant growth produce world war fast and slow. It is not only anticapitalist scholars who knew this—John Maynard Keynes himself knew it, but believed coordination and cooperation could keep growth and stability going. Government deficit spending in times of downturns, so-called countercyclical spending, was his solution to the inevitable problem of what bourgeoise economists euphemistically call the "business cycle," the fact of capital's instability. The basic and now obvious fact that endless growth cannot coexist with life on a living and finite planet, evokes the refrain repeated by economists, an inadvertent confession of the discipline's time-horizon: *in the short-run, you gotta be a Keynesian, because in the long-run, we're all dead.* The pageantry of securing the insatiable world disorder's economic infrastructure relies on providing the illusion of assured dependability in a future that must forever be staved off, all the while, the destruction performed today in the name of this charade produces a certain future no one would choose if given the choice.

In a sense, the neoliberal turn ushered in a prolonged and constant world war that happened underneath the noses of the populations of the so-called Western democratic world. The changes ushered in during this era are often shrugged off as matters of technological advancement or the progressive march of modernity, but like earlier phases of imperialism, global finance and global security concerns (the capacity to wage and win wars to secure the purse) drove the mutation of the Bretton Woods world order beyond recognition and increasingly in ways that didn't align with the official concepts of who was in charge and which borders and other manmade and taken-for-granted conventions mattered or for whom.

Given Keynes' prescience in predicting the economic and social fallout from the Treaty of Versailles and the resulting Second World War, he was given a leadership role in the twenty-two-day postwar conference held at Bretton Woods, New Hampshire, officially called the United Nations Monetary and Financial Conference. Under Keynes' intellectual guidance, Bretton Woods saw the introduction of global monetary coordination, the linchpin of which was the dollar-to-gold pegged system, wherein other countries were meant to fix their national currency's exchange rate, no longer to metal, but to the US dollar, which would be fixed to gold at the price of $35 an ounce. This was an attempt to correct for the gold standard's inherent deflationary impulse, which, in tethering the value of money to the metal, constrained the amount of growth possible to the amount of gold in the world economic system, as well as to prevent the competitive currency devaluations and resulting destabilization that plagued Europe in the periods before both world wars.

Keynes set out to save capitalism from its internal crisis problems as an effort to stave off the resulting, baked-in tendency of the system to devolve into warfare. Keynesianism's tenuous compromise, the shared gains of warfare-driven prosperity that produced the economic base for the "Thirty Glorious Years" of economic growth and relatively good terms for the working class in the industrial, imperialist core, began to sputter out by the early seventies. The emergence of OPEC and resulting price shocks led to double-digit inflation, and the Philips curve, the long-assumed axiom of an inherent tradeoff between inflation and unemployment, a barometer for Keynesian-prescribed "countercyclical" fiscal policy, no longer held.

The "stagflation" crisis—stagnation (low GDP growth and high unemployment) and high inflation—created a sense of urgency for a new economic policy and paved the way for the coup of class power that became the neoliberal revolution. Keynes's stories of balanced growth and cooperation lost sway in favor of a renewed emphasis on "pure" economic liberalism. Highlighting the "breaking" of the Phillips Curve to debunk the Keynesian orthodoxy of state intervention in the market, capitalist class agents seized on the ideological crisis in policy to promote the agenda of deregulation organized around "free market" logics.

The neoliberal fix was sold as bootstraps *self-reliance*, playing into notions of individuality and individual freedoms. In an effort to provoke the working class against the idea of organizing as a class, overt and covert campaigns capitalized on instances of union corruption to suggest that unions, rather than capitalists and corporations, are a parasitic force of no use to the individual worker enterprising enough to "think for himself." Coopting the rebelliousness of the revolutionary spirit of 1968, the neoliberal moment sought to sell a libertarian self-determination bent to the countercultural ethos. The notion was to produce a new generation of voters buying into a society of the individual, bucking planning and social cooperation as limits to freedom. The project painted the unregulated market as the source of freedom, playing against a foil of Soviet-style tyranny.

Capitalist and capitalist-state crises articulate in formations summoned into being in accordance with the saleable narrative and resultant policy approaches that directed the "fix" for the preceding crisis.[5] Neoliberal politicians, economists and other class agents sold the American public on the destruction of social welfare benefits by promising that the so-called free market, if sufficiently unbridled from the cumbersome inefficiencies of state interventions, would provide work to anyone who truly wanted it. Unions were busted and collective bargaining outlawed in accordance with the argument that they distorted the so-called free market's magic, creating an 'unfair' balance of power between employers and workers, and were the culprit behind persistently high inflation.

DEPARTURE FROM THE REAL—THE FIAT, FLOATING FINANCIALIZED REGIME

In an attempt to bail the country out of a severe balance of payments crisis and deepening economic recession, US President Richard Nixon suspended the gold-dollar peg in 1971, effectively ending the Bretton Woods global fixed monetary regime. This thrust the dollar and the rest of the world's currencies into a fiat, credit-money regime. Bullion-backed monetary regimes are inherently deflationary. Growth is constrained because it is bound to the amount of the available metallic base. Trade wars, competitive currency devaluations and reminting projects abound in the history of the making of the modern economic (dis)order, typically coincident with war-time eruptions, all of which represents attempts to resolve balance of payments and liquidity

---

5. David Harvey, "Crises of Capitalism," *RSA Animate*, September 3, 2009, https://www.youtube.com/watch?v=qOP2V_np2c0.

problems, the limits to circulation and ongoing growth in imperi-al-cum-national economic regimes.[6]

The long project of capitalist class capture—known as "deregu-lation"—allowed for several key emergences that shaped production, social reproduction, and the facts of life in the neoliberal dis-order: the proliferation of anonymous and politically active forces shaping policy at every scale; the farfetched notion of the self-policing corpo-ration while intensifying the state policing of poor and working-class people and especially, Black and Brown people and activist groups; the intensification of the rate of profit through the increased exploitation of labor, as precarious and degraded conditions enabled capitalists to squeeze more surplus value from value-producing laborers. It also ushered in additional extractivist tactics for growth: increased foreign direct investment (FDI) and state capture allowed for more mining and gas operations, capitalist-class tax dodging and state austerity log-ics, and the expansion of debt-based, finance-sector backed dysposses-sion and rentier exploitation.

The neoliberal turn was conjured into being as if it was a logical advance in thought, an enlightened way of conducting human-envi-ronment relations, when really this new take simply allowed social needs to be more totally subsumed into the market's desires. Hav-ing diagnosed regulatory red tape and working-class power as the barriers to capital's growth, the neoliberal revolution took hold not through evidence on the claim, but through sentiment and sound-bites. In his 2001 book, *Workfare States*, Jamie Peck makes an appeal for more scholarship on understanding the neoliberal state appara-tus, and in particular, implores scholars to help elucidate how and why neoliberal governance and policies travel so fast, are adapted and adopted, across place and context, so swiftly. In my estimation, to a large extent this is because neoliberal ideology so successfully detaches governance from *the real*. The project succeeded in reform-ing not only governance but our way of seeing and knowing. The neoliberal era's dismantling of Keynesian and Progressive-era state regulations meant to safeguard the wealthy, imperialist core from the worst of the system's tactics for growth amounted to an advertising

---

6.　Barry Eichengreen, *Globalizing Capital: A History on the International Monetary System* (Leuven: Leuven University Press, 1996).

sales pitch, a campaign to change what Gramsci called common sense. Academic knowledge was cherry-picked and contorted in support of the forgone policy direction, as in the Cartesian era of imperial expansion. The same tactics of focusing on abstraction, representation, and discourse were used to create a sea change in statecraft and citizenry, while the material base, the conditions and means of survival, were eroded and weaponized.

Neoliberalism is about the story that can be spun on a backdrop of depoliticized data, occluding from view the question of what is and is not measured and counted. Under neoliberalism's logic, policy is buttressed by strict focus on growth metrics, aggregate performance snapshots, evidence constructed to sell the project amidst vast landscapes of increasing social abandonment and encroaching unmet human need. Put more simply, neoliberal policies travel well because these policies are sold publicly as technocratic and rational "management," based on supposedly neutral and objective "data," omitting more complex and damning realities of daily existence for individuals and the collective. The countervailing Soviet example contributed to the villainization of the very notion of planning, including of social goods and goals, such as environmental welfare, public health, and state involvement in industrial innovation and strategy.[7] The disavowal of "state intervention," a political ideal more than a policy in practice, fostered changes in the collection, measurement, utilization, and presentation of data. Under the auspices of being hands-off, and pro-market, all manner of national reporting abandoned place-based, long-term, collective considerations in favor of rationales and political practices that cherry picked, reconfigured, abolished the collection of, misrepresented and weaponized data, instantiating the emergence of a system of governance deploying what data scientist Cathy O'Neil calls *weapons of math destruction*.[8]

Deregulation, the digital revolution, and other technological advances such as containerized shipping, combined with the decoupling of the dollar from a metallic base allowed capital the freedom to take flight from its former marriage to three-dimensional spacetime,

---

7.   Clyde V. Prestowitz, *Three Billion New Capitalists: The Great Shift of Wealth and Power to the East* (New York: Basic Books, 2006).

8.   Cathy O'Neil, *Weapons of Math Destruction: How Big Data Increases Inequality and Threatens Democracy* (New York: Crown Publishing Group, 2016).

economic life lived in place. Discourse, image, representation and sales pitches stood in for sound policy and transparency at all scales of institutional decision making. Michael Lewis, in his shocking account of Wall Street's post-2008 race to adopt high-speed and algorithmic trading, *Flash Boys*, offers one snapshot of the extent of the heist. In a meeting room an investment bank executive is negotiating a deal with a company primed to revolutionize asset trading by selling access to the fastest possible internet cable between the Chicago Mercantile Exchange and Wall Street, essentially allowing brokerage firms to receive customer orders in time to trade against them first—something that is by now common practice. The executive, from Citigroup in this instance, expressed definitive enthusiasm for the plan, but offered caution about the wording of the contract. Heeding that it would need to support "plausible deniability" by skirting the nature of the endeavor, he quips, "*It's all about optics.*"[9] In another frank admission, private equity giant Blackstone's credit division GSO came under scrutiny for a maneuver it invented in 2013 known as a "manufactured default." The practice involves offering a firm financial incentive to default on its debt in order that GSO's fund can cash in on derivative side bets, a short against the debt. In 2017 they persuaded US homebuilding firm Hovnanian to do just this, but the deal was halted after public scrutiny. Incoming head of GSO said about the incident, "We learnt a very hard lesson; we underestimated the public nature of that transaction."[10]

Deregulation has allowed for shell games, accounting tricks, and the formidable and clandestine class power of shadow, offshore and anonymized actors, often pursuing state-backed payouts or bailouts. In an investigative report on the pervasive practice of parking capital into luxury condos and other real estate, as anonymized stores of wealth, *The New York Times* found that over half of all residential real estate purchases in New York City for properties valued at more than $5 million were purchased by anonymous buyers using shell companies, unidentifiable trusts and limited liability corporations. US laws

9.   Michael Lewis, *Flash Boys: A Wall Street Revolt* (New York: W. W. Norton & Company, 2014).
10.   Robert Smith and Mark Vandevelde, "Blackstone's GSO Wrestles with Its Future," *Financial Times*, December 20, 2019, https://www.ft.com/content/4b7dbb3e-21cb-11ea-b8a1-584213ee7b2b.

allow for such transactions to take place with virtually untraceable money. "As an indication of how well-cloaked shell company owner-ship is, it took *The New York Times* more than a year to unravel the ownership of shell companies with condos in the Time Warner Cen-ter, by searching business and court records from more than twenty countries, interviewing dozens of people with close knowledge of the complex, examining hundreds of property records and connecting the dots from lawyers or relatives named on deeds to the actual buyers."[11] Researchers from the International Monetary Fund and the Univer-sity of Copenhagen reported in a September 2019 publication that 40 percent of global foreign direct investment flows were "phantom capi-tal," accounting measures in the service of tax dodging.[12] In addition to dark pools, shell companies, shadow banking, and the like, one indi-cation of the degree of fiction and fraud in the financial system is the ubiquity of the practice known as "regulatory arbitrage," squeezing profits and riding razor-thin liquidity margins by willfully disobeying what limited regulation has been kept in place in the finance sector.[13]

That the individual, *Homo economicus*, is the champion of the sys-tem's animating logic, yet chooses to act clandestinely, bears a telling contradiction. Today capital moves in inconceivable sums in the frac-tion of the time it takes to blink an eye. Its agents are also cunning and adept at coopting critique and constructing saleable lies with very lit-tle, if any, consequences. In controlling the means of knowledge pro-duction and media dissemination, the capitalist class captured greater depths of our collective sense of what's real, reasonable, and for the good of all.

11. Louise Story and Stephanie Saul, "Stream of Foreign Wealth Flows to Elite New York Real Estate," *New York Times*, February 7, 2015, sec. New York, https://www.nytimes.com/2015/02/08/nyregion/stream-of-foreign-wealth-flows-to-time-warner-condos.html.

12. Jannick Damgaard, Thomas Elkjaer, and Niels Johanssesen, "The Rise of Phantom FDI in Global Tax Havens – IMF F&D," Finance and Development (International Monetary Fund, September 2019), https://www.imf.org/external/pubs/ft/fandd/2019/09/the-rise-of-phantom-FDI-in-tax-havens-damgaard.htm.

13. John Plender, "The Seeds of the Next Debt Crisis," *Financial Times*, March 4, 2020, https://www.ft.com/content/27cf0690-5c9d-11ea-b0ab-339c2307bcd4; John McDermott, "The Where and What of Regulatory Arbitrage," *Financial Times Alphaville*, March 9, 2011, http://ftalphaville.ft.com/2011/03/09/509146/the-where-and-what-of-regulatory-arbitrage/; Caro-line Binham, Delphine Strauss, and Chris Giles, "FCA Probes Eavesdropping at Bank of England Press Conferences," *Financial Times*, December 19, 2019, https://www.ft.com/content/e5e1daea-21f6-11ea-92da-f0c92e957a96.

The 1990s saw even greater seismic shifts in the global economy that went largely undetected in the mainstream narratives of the "end of history," the collapse of the Soviet economic model and the transformation of the Chinese economy into a totalitarian capitalist regime integrated into world markets. The massive coming online of Sino and post-Soviet capital into the global pool of money, all the world's capital hungrily chasing a return, coincided with sweeping deregulation in financial, banking, real estate, environmental and labor laws that were touted as commonsense improvements aiding the supposed ease of "doing business."[14] As any of the countless scandals, such as the Panama and Paradise papers, belie, the move succeeded in its intention to make the global capitalist class's actors and actions impossible to trace. In the simplistic logic of the neoliberal sales pitch (*freedom equals free markets; states are 'inefficient' and bad; markets are 'efficient' and therefore good*) trans- and post-national backroom deals and alliances became convention, and the capitalist class pursued its always-global ambitions, including the capture of state and multilateral institutions. This phenomenon in the US is partly evident in the obvious revolving door phenomena of corporate executives into governmental regulatory roles—at the FDA, the Departments Agriculture, Education, and Defense, as well as the symbiotic relationship between Wall Street and the Treasury Department. This is part and parcel to what David Harvey has named the "State-Finance Nexus."

The post-1971 financial turn promised that a democratization of capital, or rather the extension of debts to more people for more things, would be a springboard for opportunity and economic growth. Debts, public and private, proliferated and soared in the forty-year period. According to the Institute for International Finance, debt to GDP ratios globally reached an all-time high in the third quarter of 2019, measuring more than 322 percent.[15] As the privilege to become indebted was extended to more people for the fulfilment of increasingly basic needs, the state did its part by revising debtor laws to favor creditors, simultaneously repealing usury laws while drastically curtailing the legal circumstances under which borrowers could be

14.   See World Bank's Doing Business Report 2004–2020, https://archive.doingbusiness.org/en/doingbusiness.
15.   Plender, "The Seeds of the Next Debt Crisis."

exempted from debt contracts, no matter how predatory. Historian Ellen Meiksins Wood's observation that the historiography of capitalism's origins conflates the compulsion to participate in the system with 'opportunity,' is useful for understanding how the agents of the neoliberal turn systematically used the language of rights, opportunity, and inclusion to promote the intensification of capitalist-growth oriented social formations at every scale of life.[16]

THE GOLPE GROWTH REGIME
AND THE EMBODIED SPATIAL FIX

Reformist Keynesians emphasize the reckless and criminal tactics of the so-called cowboy capitalist ethos of the neoliberal era. They drum on the irresponsible behavior of hedge funds and private equity firms whose risk-to-reward calculations are more extreme than the more measured or 'conservative' approach of pension and other long-term fund managers. Yet for all this emphasis, it is the benign-seeming interest-bearing savings and investment accounts, retirement savings chiefly among them, seeking a modest (historically, until very recently, a steady three percent) rate of return, that, in the perpetually slowed growth climate of the last decades with its record-low interest rates on government bonds, drives the madness of such financial logic. One well-known example is the subprime scandal. The slowed growth climate has also driven more pension funds and conservative investment portfolios into the arms of private equity firms, whose twenty percent fees and unscrupulous pump-and-dump strategies have been one of the only yield-bearing games in town. Financial tactics in the derivative and reinsurance markets put the public's wealth on the hook in three-card-monte style trade configurations, where the state and the working class very well may lose, but the house always wins.[17] Debt-backed asset bubbles, fueled by cheap borrowing and perpetual quantitative easing, turned to cashed-out gains for the asset-owning class

---

16.   Ellen Meiksins Wood, "The Non-History of Capitalism," *Historical Materialism* 1, no. 1 (January 1, 1997): 5–21; Ellen Meiksins Wood, *The Origin of Capitalism: A Longer View* (New York and London: Verso, 2002).

17.   The card game reference is from my friend Raymond Luc Levasseur's unpublished essay "Requiem for Albert Glaude" (2017).

and ever more entrapping networks of paying and borrowing to live for the wage-dependent working class. And because the money being played with amounts to no less than all the world's savings, everyone with a pension fund or investment account is implicated. Capital grows in the name of working-class people's retirement accounts by dispossessing working-class people of their homes.

Neoliberalism was a global *golpe*. By untying gold from the dollar, capital's limits could defy its spacetime contract with the Earth. This was the equivalent of a sonic rupture, piercing the fabric of our known reality. Wall Street's arrangement with newly empowered oil-producing regimes set young bankers out on the task of recycling petrodollars around the world, inspiring CIA-backed coups and high debt burdens in the name of something called "economic development" in the rest of the underdeveloped world.

Neoliberalism turned the American blue-collar working class into *tierra firma*, a spatial fix through which to circulate capital. Capital no longer needed a mass of industrial, working-class laborers in the heartland of the empire. Reconfigurations via outsourcing, offshoring, labor-saving technology and streamlined global logistics allowed the bulk of industrial production to be done by much more heavily exploited laborers in other parts of the world. Instead, what it needed was territory through which capital could circulate and valorize, to stave off overaccumulation crises. Through pills, prison, mortgages, student, medical and other kinds of consumer debt, the global economic disorder reconfigured the American blue-collar working class as conduits, territory from which to extract profit. In *Golden Gulag*, Ruth Wilson Gilmore articulates what she calls the "prison fix." The elucidation, along with Harvey's foundation of the spatial fix, allows us to see the pain pill fix.[18]

To contain the resultant social fallout, the empire resorted to violence, suppression, geographical containment, isolation, and extermination. Neoliberalism was sold in public discourse as a solution to supposed state inefficiencies, but in reality, neoliberalism has instead produced what geographer Ruth Wilson Gilmore remarks is a

---

18. The concept of the spatial fix is elaborated in Chapter 5.

meaner, but not leaner, state.[19] The delegitimization of social welfare and the subsequent gutting of Keynesian state formations has produced what Gilmore and others calls the "shadow state," or the "anti-state state," which is to say political and state formations that purport to be *noninterventionist*.[20]

In a talk in Washington Square Park during Occupy Wall Street, David Graeber put the matter succinctly: "Financialization is a euphemism for militarization. The mechanisms are meant to be obscured."[21] As he argued in his book *Debt*, debt-based (fiat) regimes are backed by the state's power to reduce human beings to not only consumers or conduits, but to money itself.[22]

Displaced former and would-be laborers, whose numbers soared in the neoliberal era, become valuable in capital's image precisely for the fact of their dispossession and social devaluation. The displaced formerly working class bolster the ranks of the so-called reserve army of surplus labor against whom working people's wages can be bid down, allowing for higher rates of exploitation of the working class. They also, through state and market-based fixes that produce from surplussed people new circuits of consumption and accumulation, solve the problem of effective demand. State and market actors invent new channels, means and logics through which capital can affix, transfix, and transform, through and in the name of surplus populations, allowing for growth, principal plus interest, the return of profit.

Incarceration, disability, Medicare cards, pain pills—all of these state-capital infrastructures allow capital to flow, in the name of new and old logics that do not attempt to resolve capitalism's produced social problems but capital's inherent crises of circulation, exchange and profitability. Prisons and pain pills resolve crises of capital. In these circuits, capitalism's constant conundrum of needing to both squeeze the share of profits going to labor and its need for consumers, is *fixed* by the carceral state in the first instance, and by the state- or

19.   Ruth Wilson Gilmore, *Golden Gulag: Prisons, Surplus, Crisis, and Opposition in Globalizing California* (Oakland: University of California Press, 2007), 53.

20.   Ruth Wilson Gilmore, "Globalisation and US Prison Growth: From Military Keynesianism to Post-Keynesian Militarism," *Race and Class* 40, no. 2–3 (1999).

21.   Personal notes, David Graeber's *Debt the First* 5,000 *Years* book talk in Washington Square Park, April 2012.

22.   David Graeber, *Debt: The First 5,000 Years* (Brooklyn and London: Melville House, 2011), 171.

private- (insurance or out-of-pocket) funded consumption of addictive opioids in the last. Despite a lack of working-class purchasing power, prisons and pain pills produce a compulsion to consume. Highly addictive opioids, especially when paid for by third-party state or private insurance, help solve the problem of effective demand for a capitalist class that has, over the past forty years, decimated labor's capacity to get/buy. This represents an organized circuit of capital accumulation, channeling through socially and physically displaced human beings—who may once have been organized into labor unions. In turning working and would-be working people into "addicts" seeking a fix, capital, the real fiend, finds the fix it cannot live without.

BREAKING LABOR'S BACK

Neoliberalism brought about the structural abandonment of the American blue-collar working class. Union membership rates were at their peak in the US in 1954, at 35 percent of the labor force. In the 1970s, the number was still around 33 percent of all workers. In 2023, only 10 percent of the labor force is unionized.[23] Unions didn't only provide bargaining power but were central to working-class community. They were fraternal organizations and a significant source of political education and class-based social analysis. The decimation of organized labor eroded both infrastructure for communal belonging and the economic purchasing power requisite for anything like leisure time. As disposable income eroded, local businesses that served as recreation and gathering places closed.

All of this is a familiar enough story, evocative in the title of political scientist Robert Putnam's 2000 book *Bowling Alone*. The story is also told on the landscape of the former-industrial-cum-Rust Belt, whose abandoned factories frame decimated shells of once lively working-class communities. In short order, the blue-collar worker went from enjoying the fruits of their labor to being isolated and in fear. "*Ten years burning down the road*," as the Boss [Bruce Springsteen] sung it, "*Ain't got nowhere to run, nowhere to go.*"

---

23. Dee-Ann Durbin, "US Unions Flexed Their Muscles Last Year, but Membership Rates Fall to All-Time Low," *AP News*, January 23, 2024, https://apnews.com/article/unions-membership-rates-uaw-government-a3fc7bc50dd59a89f414230e8837d7e6.

Proponents of financial deregulation often speak of the trade-offs between "short-run pain" for "long-run gain." With no regard for distributional effects (spatiality and dimensional difference), stock-index aggregates and econometric modeling evidenced the supposed net goodness of financial liberalization the world over. When distribution is factored, of course, a clear pattern emerges demonstrating with specificity *whose* pain means *whose* gain.

Thomas Piketty and Gabriel Zucman, using an augmented long-run, multinational macroeconomic database—which inspired Piketty's *Capital in the 21st Century* (2017)—assert that global wealth imbalances have reached levels not seen since the early days of industrialization. In other words, "Capital is Back."[24] In 2019 the Federal Reserve released a new composite index, the Distributional Financial Accounts, comprising two long-time longitudinal datasets, the Financial Accounts or "Flow of Funds," (z1) dataset and the Survey of Consumer Finances.[25] The time series stretch from 1989 to 2018. Among the many interesting insights present in the data, one summary statistic stands out: over the timespan covered, net wealth gains by the wealthiest 1 percent of Americans increased by a total of $21 trillion, while the bottom 50 percent saw a combined net wealth decrease of $900 billion.[26] An analysis of the data by the People's Policy Project found that present-day inequality in the United States is at its worst point since the 1920s, and by way of illustration offered a striking datapoint: In 2019, the three wealthiest people in America had as much wealth as the bottom 50 percent.[27]

Precarious circumstances predominate American working-class life. A 2018 report by the Urban Institute found that 40 percent of American households struggled to afford basic needs, leading David Lazarus to declare in the title of an *LA Times* column, "The Economy

24. Thomas Piketty and Gabriel Zucman, "Capital Is Back: Wealth-Income Ratios in Rich Countries 1700–2010," *The Quarterly Journal of Economics* 129, no. 3 (August 2014): 1255–1310.
25. Michael M. Batty et al., "Introducing the Distributional Financial Accounts of the United States," Finance and Economics Discussion Series (Board of Governors of the Federal Reserve System (US), March 22, 2019), https://ideas.repec.org/p/fip/fedgfe/2019-17.html.
26. Board of Governors of the Federal Reserve System, "Financial Accounts of the United States – Z.1 Release," November 23, 2018, https://www.federalreserve.gov/releases/z1/20181206/html/index.htm.
27. Matt Bruenig, "Top 1% Up $21 Trillion. Bottom 50% Down $900 Billion," People's Policy Project, October 9, 2019, https://www.peoplespolicyproject.org/2019/06/14/top-1-up-21-trillion-bottom-50-down-900-billion/.

May Be Booming but Nearly Half of Americans Can't Make Ends Meet."[28] A CDC report in 2018 concluded that 19 million Americans faced housing insecurity, attributable to stagnant wages and "soaring" housing costs. Rising disability rosters is another measure of displaced would-be blue-collar workers. According to a 2018 Congressional Research Service report, the total number of people receiving disability was about 2.7 million in 1985. As of December 2017, 8.7 million people were on the rosters, after having peaked at 9 million people in 2014. The declining rate is due in part to the passage of the Affordable Care act and also the political maneuvering to make disability more difficult to obtain in response to backlash at the sharply rising rolls.[29]

THE PAIN PILL FIX

Journalist: Do you think the doctor that prescribes you pills knows that you're addicted?
Respondent: Yes. For sure.
Journalist: Why do you think he still prescribes you pills?
Respondent: Because he wants money.

—*The OxyContin Express* (Vanguard TV, 2009)

The opioid crisis was produced according to capital's logic and is one among countless articulations of capitalism's endemic pattern of producing plunder and pain for the sake of profit. Like all drug epidemics, the opioid epidemic is a predominantly supply-side induced phenomenon. The competitive drive for profits in the deregulated, for-profit medicine schema, in the context of widescale neoliberal state capture, collided with the embodied pain of the economically displaced and dispossessed American working class.

Capital competes for profit margins across sectors. As intensification in the rate of profit accelerated in the finance sector, the pharmaceutical sector also pursued intensification and extractivist tactics.

28. David Lazarus, "The Economy May Be Booming, but Nearly Half of Americans Can't Make Ends Meet," *Los Angeles Times*, August 31, 2018, https://www.latimes.com/business/lazarus/la-fi-lazarus-economy-stagnant-wages-20180831-story.html.
29. Terrence McCoy, "Disabled or Just Desperate? Rural Americans Turn to Disability as Jobs Dry Up," *Washington Post*, March 30, 2017, https://www.washingtonpost.com/sf/local/2017/03/30/disabled-or-just-desperate/.

The finance sector's innovations in speed and intensity of extracted gains sets the bar for other capitalist class actors. *Short-term, high-yield* became an organizing principle for all sectors of capitalist class actors, permeating all of life with an extractivist ethos that is against life itself. Thus as the deregulated financial industry began operating under more elaborate and dodgy tactics like using shell companies, dark pools, and other accounting and regulatory tricks, pharma's use of similar tactics also intensified. In a for-profit medical system in general and particularly amidst the ever-more pervasive investment climate of *short-term, high-yield*, pharma has become a highly lucrative growth engine in the American economy. McKinsey and Company report that the healthcare sector has the highest returns to shareholders of any sector, outstripping consumer staples, energy, or tech.[30] Amidst all the remarking of the postindustrial era's penchant for financial over manufacturing investments in the neoliberal restructuring to what David Harvey calls the flexible regime of accumulation, the pharmaceutical industry, which still makes a tangible commodity in a factory, has the highest profit margin of any sector in the American economy.

NERVOUS SYSTEMS: BENZOS AND COMMODIFIED RELIEF

The story of how drugs like Valium and Xanax became household names cannot be told without mentioning the Sackler family's narco-philanthropic empire. Until very recently it was not uncommon to see mentions of the Sackler family name in laudatory terms, totally disconnected from the facts of how they made their fortune. Thanks to some eventual investigative reports and a growing direct-action protest movement, the connection between the family name and the opioid epidemic is now finally explicit.[31]

30.　Ralf Otto, Alberto Santagostino, and Ulf Schrader, "Rapid Growth in Biopharma: Challenges and Opportunities | Mckinsey & Company," June 14, 2018, https://www.mckinsey.com/industries/pharmaceuticals-and-medical-products/our-insights/rapid-growth-in-biopharma.
31.　Direct actions at the Guggenheim and the Louvre in the summer of 2019 coordinated by organizers with the groups Sackler PAIN and Decolonize This Place gained widespread attention and resulted in the Louvre removing the Sackler name from their buildings. Shortly after, the Metropolitan Museum of Art, the Guggenheim Museum, and other arts institutions stated that they would no longer accept donations from the family. See David Armstrong, "Inside Purdue Pharma's Media Playbook: How It Planted the Opioid 'Anti-Story,'" *ProPublica*, November 19, 2019, https://www.propublica.org/article/

Brothers Arthur and Mortimer Sackler were the founding partners of what would become the Sackler pharma empire. Both brothers attended medical school, with Arthur specializing in psychiatry before attending business school where he earned a degree in marketing. In 1952, Arthur purchased a small-time, mostly laxative producing, drug company named Purdue Frederick, which later became Purdue Pharmaceuticals with the revenue he earned selling the drug Terramycin for Pfizer. Arthur founded his own pharmaceutical advertising firm the same year.

Arthur Sackler, everyone says, revolutionized the field of pharmaceutical advertising. In the same year he bought Purdue and opened his own ad firm, he became the first ad man to convince *The Journal of the American Medical Association*, the most well-regarded publication in the profession, to allow for the placement of a color "advertorial" brochure.[32] During Arthur's lifetime, the family-owned ad firm did not handle the marketing launches of Purdue drugs.[33] The launch of OxyContin in 1996 would be the first handled directly by the family firm and it was overseen by Arthur's nephew Richard Sackler.

Forty years before their prominent role in mainstreaming opioid use, the Sacklers played a crucial role in making benzodiazepines a common factor of American life. Arthur Sackler's role in the campaign to make Valium a household name forewarned the family strategy of blending medicine and marketing. The story of benzodiazepines begins with first accidental discovery in a pharmaceutical laboratory in 1955 of chlordiazepoxide (Librium), which was patented and marketed by Hoffmann-La Roche in 1960. Hoffmann-La Roche hired Arthur Sackler's advertising firm to launch the campaign for Librium. A few years later, another chemical cousin was discovered, biologically identical

inside-purdue-pharma-media-playbook-how-it-planted-the-opioid-anti-story; Harriet Ryan, Lisa Girion, and Scott Glover, "'You Want a Description of Hell?' OxyContin's 12-Hour Problem #InvestigatingOxy," *Los Angeles Times*, May 6, 2016, http://www.latimes.com/projects/OxyContin-part1/; Scott Higham et al., "76 Billion Opioid Pills: Newly Released Federal Data Unmasks the Epidemic," *Washington Post*, December 3, 2019, https://www.washingtonpost.com/investigations/76-billion-opioid-pills-newly-released-federal-data-unmasks-the-epidemic/2019/07/16/5f29fd62-a73e-11e9-86dd-d7f0e60391e9_story.html; Patrick Radden Keefe, "The Family That Built an Empire of Pain," *New Yorker*, October 23, 2017, https://www.newyorker.com/magazine/2017/10/30/the-family-that-built-an-empire-of-pain.

32. Christopher Glazek, "The Secretive Family Making Billions from the Opioid Crisis," *Esquire*, October 16, 2017, https://www.esquire.com/news-politics/a12775932/sackler-family-OxyContin/.

33. Arthur Sackler died on May 26, 1987.

in its action on the human organism but molecularly distinct enough to earn Hoffmann-La Roche a separate patent and therefore a new product line. It named this second drug Valium. The 1963 rollout and marketing campaign for Valium is widely considered a game changing marketing campaign, touted as pharma's "first modern advertising campaign," a phrase that would be echoed by the Sackler family's own blockbuster drug OxyContin's marketing campaign in 1996.[34]

While Valium was virtually indistinguishable from Librium, Sackler promoted Valium by "audaciously inflating its range of indications."[35] While Librium was marketed as a treatment for garden-variety anxiety, Sackler positioned Valium as an elixir for a problem he christened "psychic tension." "According to his ads, psychic tension, the forebear of today's colloquially ubiquitous 'stress,' was the secret culprit behind a host of somatic conditions, including heartburn, gastrointestinal issues, insomnia, and restless-leg syndrome."[36]

Sackler's marketing efforts turned the tranquilizers Librium and Valium into everyday commodities. In the 1960s, Valium became the top-prescribed drug in the nation and the first pharmaceutical to reach $100 million in sales. One particularly impactful advertisement for Valium, which appeared in medical trade publications showed a full-page closeup of a woman's distressed face, gritting her teeth, in a grimace, and with a furrowed brow. Inside the image were several gradually smaller images of the same woman's face settling into progressively more calm states, and looking content, or at least placated and a little glazed over, by the last image. In large lettering across the top of the page read the words, "reduce psychic tension."

Valium would earn the moniker "Mother's Little Helper," popularized by the 1966 Rolling Stones song of the same name. The Stones' song captures the general sentiment of the drug. Valium takes the edges off the everyday discomforts of an unfulfilling life, and offers relief for the build-up of tension associated not with acute stress but with the cumulative stresses of seemingly mundane dis-ease:

---

34. Art Van Zee, "The Promotion and Marketing of OxyContin: Commercial Triumph, Public Health Tragedy," *American Journal of Public Health* 99, no. 2 (February 2009): 221–227.
35. Glazek, "The Secretive Family Making Billions from the Opioid Crisis."
36. Glazek, "The Secretive Family Making Billions from the Opioid Crisis."

What a drag it is getting old
'Kids are different today,'
I hear ev'ry mother say
Mother needs something today to calm her down
And though she's not really ill
There's a little yellow pill
She goes running for the shelter of a mother's little helper
And it helps her on her way, gets her through her busy day

Like opioids, physiological tolerance to benzos builds quickly as does psychological habituation. *"Doctor please, some more of these. Outside the door, she took four more,"* the song continues.

By 1973, millions of annual tranquilizer prescriptions had created what Senator Edward Kennedy bewailed as a "a nightmare of dependence and addiction.[37] By 1977 benzos were the most widely prescribed class of drugs worldwide, with Valium being one of the top five most prescribed drugs in the US throughout the seventies. In 1984, at an average US price of .30 cents for a 5-milligram pill, 25 million prescriptions for Valium were written, and Hoffmann-La Roche grossed more than $240 million in sales from the drug, making Valium the then-highest grossing drug in history.[38]

PROFIT AND INCENTIVE STRUCTURES IN PHARMA

Valium normalized the notion of the pervasiveness of low-level and chronic mood disorders as a modern fact of life, for which drugs could help. In putting Swiss drug maker Hoffman-La Roche on the map in the US pharma landscape, the commercial success of Valium paved the way for other pharmaceutical companies to focus their growth strategies on psychiatric, mood, and chronic tension disorders.

The now-ubiquitous notion of pharmaceutical "patent cliffs" was ushered into being by the passage of the 1984 Drug Price Competition

---

37. Sam Pizzigati, "The Big Pharama Family that Brought Us the Opioid Crisis," *Inequality.org*, February 16, 2018, https://inequality.org/great-divide/big-pharma-firm-brought-us-opioid-crisis/.
38. Marlene Cimons, "U.S. Expected to Allow Sale of Generic Valium," *Los Angeles Times*, September 4, 1985, http://articles.latimes.com/1985-09-04/business/fi-23293_1_generic-competition.

and Patent Restoration Act. The law shortened patent terms and streamlined the process for generic competitor formulations to reach market. The "cliff effect" results from the way in which the discovery, development and patenting of a new drug class typically occurs in a cohort, with different firms patenting their slightly distinct molecular formulations at around the same time. This leads whole classes of patented drugs (benzodiazepines, SSRIs, etc.) to expire at once. The "cliff" refers to this sudden loss of profitability throughout the industry. This results in herding behavior, as branded firms rush to develop the first patent in what will become the next "blockbuster" class of drugs.

"Evergreening" is a related practice used to stave off the devastation of impending patent cliffs. The term describes the convention of pharma firms getting new patents or extensions on patent rights for existing drugs in the name of slight, usually medically inconsequential, modifications to the drug. A study by the US Patent Office found that of the 100 top-selling drugs between 2005 and 2015, 80 percent had received at least one patent extension and half had received multiple extensions.[39] Another study over the same time period covering all drugs on the market found that "[r]ather than creating new medicines, pharmaceutical companies are largely recycling and repurposing old ones. Specifically, 78 percent of the drugs associated with new patents were not new drugs, but existing ones, and extending protection is particularly pronounced among blockbuster drugs."[40] Evergreening can amount to a benign tweak to a molecular structure that does not change the drug's efficacy or biological functioning at all, or, like Purdue did with its trademarked Contin mechanism, can involve applying a patented time-release mechanism to a long-existing off-patent drug, like morphine (MS Contin) and oxycodone (OxyContin). By November 2017, Purdue had been awarded patent extensions on OxyContin as a result of such maneuvers a total of thirteen times.[41]

---

39. Ed Silverman, "Keeping the Register Ringing: Many Old Drugs Have Plenty of New Patents," *STAT*, November 8, 2017, https://www.statnews.com/pharmalot/2017/11/08/patents-evergreen-exclusivity/.
40. Robin Feldman, "May Your Drug Price Be Evergreen," SSRN Scholarly Paper (Rochester, NY: Social Science Research Network, December 7, 2018), https://papers.ssrn.com/abstract=3061567.
41. Katherine Ellen Foley, "Big Pharma Is Taking Advantage of Patent Law to Keep OxyContin from Ever Dying," *Quartz*, May 25, 2018, https://qz.com/1125690/

Exclusive patent rights are afforded for new drugs for twenty years under US patent law, and the convention is adhered to in most parts of the world.[42] Firms typically patent a drug at the earliest possible moment in the development stage to keep competitors from developing their own formulation and beating them to market. The FDA approval process typically takes twelve years (though fast-track approval initiatives underway seek to change this), leaving, on average, eight years of patent coverage during which the drug can be sold. Firms use a host of legal maneuvers to block generic patent rights approval as the patent expiry looms, the ubiquitous tactic of running out the clock in petty legal battles most common among them, but evergreening tricks attempt to extend patent coverage as long as possible before engaging in courtroom appeals.

Valium signaled that the growth engine of the industry was in further developing product lines for mood disorders and the host of rising and persistent psychosomatic complaints. With patent expirations for the class of brand-name benzos coming down the pike, in the mid-eighties, Purdue pivoted its resources and product development toward narcotic pain pills. Referring to the patent cliffs for SSRIs and benzos respectively, one researcher remarked, "The marketing of Oxy-Contin (1996) and its predecessor MS Contin (1984) began at an auspicious time."[43] Purdue developed and patented Contin, a time-release delivery formulation in 1972. In 1984, a year ahead of the benzo patent cliff, Purdue released its extended-release formulation of morphine, MS Contin, mostly used in the treatment of pain related to terminal cancer, though evidence suggests the firm sought new avenues for growth. It is well documented that the trend in doctors prescribing opioids for prolonged use for chronic, non-terminal-cancer-related pain began earlier than the debut of OxyContin, but in December 1995, coincident with the SSRI patent cliff, OxyContin became the first drug approved for this purpose.

big-pharma-is-taking-advantage-of-patent-law-to-keep-OxyContin-from-ever-dying/.

42. Matthew Herper, "Solving the Drug Patent Problem," *Forbes*, May 2, 2002, https://www.forbes.com/2002/05/02/0502patents.html; Robin Feldman, "May Your Drug Price Be Ever-green," *Journal of Law and the Biosciences* 5, no. 3 (December 2018): 590–647, https://doi.org/10.1093/jlb/lsy022.

43. Charles W. Van Way, "Bashing Big Pharma," *Missouri Medicine* 116, no. 2 (2019): 80–82.

THE PAIN MANAGEMENT FIX

The Victoria and Albert Museum in London is named for the mon-archs who presided over, among other prolonged episodes of impe-rial violence, the Opium Wars. A courtyard there, unveiled in 2017, is named for the Sacklers, the family who built, as one exposé recently called it, "an empire of pain."[44] Prior to the 1980s, 10,000 years of human consensus had implored caution in the medical use of opi-oids in the relief of pain. Seeking a new engine for growth, phar-maceutical firms organized as a class to change medical knowledge and best practice on the prescribing of opioids for chronic, non-ter-minal-illness related pain. The innovations in the formulation, prescribing guidelines and marketing of narcotic painkillers in the United States beginning in the mid-1980s were a coordinated effort. Academic institutions, researchers, medical journals and profes-sional associations participated in the pharma-driven push to nor-malize opioid-based therapy for the rising problem of non-terminal illness-related chronic pain.

In the late nineteenth and early twentieth centuries, heroin was marketed as a nonaddictive alternative to morphine. The drug's inventor, Bayer Pharmaceuticals, promoted heroin as a treatment for morphine addiction. This story of a "safer" alternative repeated itself with OxyContin. The case Purdue Pharma made to the FDA for the approval of OxyContin focused on its novel formulation, the Contin time-release mechanism, which they claimed allowed for con-trolled-release dosing of oxycodone every twelve hours instead of the standard four to six hours. This was a key selling point Purdue used to argue for OxyContin's safety and efficacy in managing pain. However, in the years following the approval, it became evident that this claim was misleading. Without providing clinical trial data to substantiate it, the FDA application made the claim that this steadier disbursal of the drug "is believed to be" virtually "nonaddictive."[45]

Eight-hour time release opioids were already on the market and so the twelve-hour claim was critical to FDA patent approval. There is speculation but no official record of how and why FDA approval was

---

44. Keefe, "The Family That Built an Empire of Pain."
45. Van Zee, "The Promotion and Marketing of OxyContin"; Sam Quinones, *Dreamland: The True Tale of America's Opiate Epidemic* (New York: Bloomsbury Press, 2015).

granted despite such glaring omissions in the case. It is by now public record that the FDA official who presided over the approval process left the agency a year later for a job at Purdue, earning a salary of over $400,000 a year.[46] After reports of physicians prescribing OxyContin dosing more frequently than twelve-hours reached Purdue, the firm organized a special training with its sales force. They instructed doctors to stick by the twelve-hour dosing protocol, and suggested in the case of patients complaining that the medicine wore off before the twelve-hour interval that the dosage be upped. In one of my last conversations with my mother, who weaned herself off prescription fentanyl at the age of seventy-nine, after twenty-six years of dependency, I learned that this twelve-hour dosing problem was a part of her story in the 1990s. "You know what he did? He upped my dose." The words stung, knowing what I did about this key piece of the whole sales strategy and crisis production.

The extremely unpleasant physiological symptoms of opioid withdrawal encourage psychological and physiological dependencies on the substance. This is not an imaginary or insignificant feature of the cycle of dependency but rather a neurophysiological mechanism that changes physical circuitry of the human brain to produce thought patterns and chemical signaling that associate the deathly feeling state of withdrawal with a sense of powerlessness over the need to consume more of the commodity. Investigative reporting in 2016 from the *Los Angeles Times* revealed the "12-hour problem" as a key explanatory factor for why medical, licit users of Oxy have a high propensity for developing dependency. Peter Przekop, a neuroscientist and physician who oversees the treatment of opioid-dependent people at the Betty Ford Center in Rancho Mirage, CA, said that repeated episodes of withdrawal from OxyContin "absolutely" raise the risk that patients will develop a dependency to the medication. "You are messing with those areas of the brain that are involved in addiction, and you are going to get the person dependent on it," he said.[47]

---

46.   Raymond Bonner, "The Sackler Family, Its Fortune, and Its Dangerous Drugs," *Sydney Morning Herald*, May 17, 2021, https://www.smh.com.au/culture/books/the-sackler-family-its-fortune-and-its-dangerous-drugs-20210507-p57ps8.html.

47.   Ryan et al., "'You Want a Description of Hell?' OxyContin's 12-Hour Problem #InvestigatingOxy."

Through shell nonprofit structures masquerading as civic groups, lobbying efforts to initiate and shape the direction of congressional studies about the rise of pain, and other measures, narco-pharma capitalist class agents pursued a revolution in the treatment of the ever-growing American problem of chronic pain.[48] The tactic mirrors that of other instances of imperial encroachment, which couch the right of capitalists to expand their market share as the morally sound deliverance of freedom, help, and relief, as they simultaneously traffic in the imposition of pain.[49]

In 2015, then-President Obama regularly cited a CDC finding that four of every five surveyed heroin users report that their dependence on opioids began with prescription pharmaceuticals.[50] While illicit redistribution and consumption surely played a role in the magnitude of the crisis' geographic spread and lethal toll, the data suggest this is not the main feature of the epidemic. Between 1999 and 2013, the number of prescriptions written for opioids in the US quadrupled and in 2013, the number of legal and recorded prescriptions for opioid analgesics filled at American pharmacies amounted to enough for each person living in the United States to have a thirty-day supply. The World Health Organization reports that in 2015, the United States consumed 99 percent of the licit supply of prescription opioid pills globally.

What is less commonly known however are the constellation of related circumstances that allowed for the mass prescribing of opioids in the United States. Class-action lawsuits against drug makers began as early as 2001, and court documents and depositions (as well as guilty pleas from high-level pharma executives) contribute to a general

48.   Institute of Medicine (US) Committee on Advancing Pain Research... , "Relieving Pain in America"; Chris McGreal, *American Overdose: The Opioid Tragedy in Three Acts* (New York: PublicAffairs, 2018); Keefe, "The Family That Built an Empire of Pain"; Julia Lurie, "'Behave More Sexually:' How Big Pharma Used Strippers, Guns, and Cash to Push Opioids," *Mother Jones*, December 6, 2019, https://www.motherjones.com/politics/2018/05/insys-subsys-whistleblower-lawsuits/; *Commonwealth of Massachusetts v. Purdue Pharma L.P., Purdue Pharma Inc., Richard Sackler, Theresa Sackler, et. al.*, January 31, 2019.
49.   David Harvey, *A Brief History of Neoliberalism* (New York: Oxford University Press, 2007); Ananya Roy, *Poverty Capital: Microfinance and the Making of Development* (London: Routledge, 2010).
50.   Obama White House, "FACT SHEET: Obama Administration Announces Public and Private Sector Efforts to Address Prescription Drug Abuse and Heroin Use," October 21, 2015, https://obamawhitehouse.archives.gov/the-press-office/2015/10/21/fact-sheet-obama-administration-announces-public-and-private-sector.

notion of corporate malfeasance, greed, and the other presumptions an under-informed but intelligent populace has deduced about the production of the crisis, but getting underneath the narrative of "a few greedy CEOs" to understand the logics and incentives that unleashed OxyContin and its cousins onto the American healthcare landscape in the mid-nineties offers important guidance for understanding the characteristics of the crisis.

THE DEMOCRATIZATION OF RELIEF

The opioid crisis was produced in a deregulated drug industry through an advertising and sales campaign that mobilized the discourse of rights and inclusion, in this case the expansion of the right to be free from pain, during a period of economic freefall rife with exponential rates of produced, embodied, socioeconomic pain. Logics of liberal inclusion proliferated in the neoliberal era, as debt-backed financial regimes required the indebtedness of more people for more rationales, the world over.

As the degraded and squeezed working class found itself ground to the bone-on-bone embodied pain of the financialized profit regime, pharma-capitalist stepped in, in a deregulated market, to offer the commodity fix for what ailed a zeitgeist—stress, depression, and pain. "Get back in the swing of things," was Purdue's marketing slogan for OxyContin, a promise to those stuck in the painful grind of falling behind, another chance, a lifeline. And while MS Contin was targeted to oncologists and for terminal cancer-related pain, OxyContin was pitched to general practitioners for a condition Purdue helped put on the map, "chronic pain." Purdue and its cohort played to the altruistic ethos of the health care professions, with sales-pitch talking points focusing on the power to be a leader in providing cutting-edge, enlightened care.[51] The marketing campaign that led to the glut of free-flowing opioid prescriptions and sales between 1996 and 2013 in the US, and that continues today in other parts of the world, cloaks the

---

51. *The Pharmacist*, directed by Jenner Furst and Julia Willoughby Nason (2020; New York: The Cinemart), Netflix.

campaign as the democratization of relief, akin to a moral mandate to expand access to narcotic pain pills.

This tactic rests on liberalism's central conceit of the 'white man's burden,' so fundamental to the development of what Ananya Roy calls *Poverty Capital* (2010), the developmentalist rationale of a "right to relief."[52] In this manner, those with opioids to sell and an interest in turning money into more money produced a sea change, a coordinated and well-funded effort to revolutionize medical common sense and produce new notions of best practice about how to treat the emerging flood of patients in American doctors' offices complaining of chronic pain. All this organizing and ground-laying was called "marketing," praised by the pharma advertising industry for being innovative and exemplary. It is more apt to regard the effort as one of *market making*: forcing changes in accepted medical knowledge and in the knowledge base, sentiment, and resultant actions and revenue circuits of medical practitioners. In changing the lay of the land in medical knowledge and best practices, Purdue and its cohort produced new territory for profit expansion. Armed with a rationale—the pain patient's right to relief—standing in for astonishingly flimsy evidence, a new claim on the old trope of a proprietary, non-habit-forming innovation of the always-habit-forming morphine molecule was made.[53] The Sackler family and other pharma firms set out to make billions from patented and generic variations of a substance that sells itself and guarantees its own ongoing, growing, demand.

THE RISE AND FALL OF A HOUSEHOLD NAME

How did the Sacklers build the 16th-largest fortune in the country? The short answer: making the most popular and controversial opioid of the 21st century—OxyContin.

—Alex Morrell, "The OxyContin Clan:The $14 Billion Newcomer to Forbes 2015 List of Richest U.S. Families," 2015[54]

52. Roy, *Poverty Capital*.
53. Quinones, *Dreamland*.
54. Alex Morrell, "The OxyContin Clan: The $14 Billion Newcomer to Forbes 2015 List of Richest U.S. Families," *Forbes*, July 1, 2015, https://www.forbes.com/sites/alexmorrell/2015/07/01/the-oxycontin-clan-the-14-billion-newcomer-to-forbes-2015-list-of-richest-u-s-families/.

Arthur Sackler's expertise was in combining psychiatry and marketing. Having engineered the Valium ad campaign popularizing pills for the treatment of his invented term "psychic tension," he may have anticipated the coming wave of embodied psychic tension that manifests as chronic physical pain.[55] Purdue's global division, headquartered in the UK and operational on four continents is, in most countries, called "Mundipharma."[56] Reuters reports the firm had $1.7 billion in annual sales in 2022.[57] On the homepage of Mundipharma's website (c. 2017), the company states: "We are an asset-led, family-owned business." "Asset-led" is a marketing term for brand-recognition, a Sackler-family ideal.

The successful branding of OxyContin is evident in the number of popular songs that reference it.[58] When the media, including *The New York Times* (2001), began reporting on the phenomenon of "The One-Pill Kill," the recalled 80 mg OxyContin tablet, or on pharmacy robberies in which masked assailants asked for OxyContin by name, leading several pharmacies in Maine to discontinue the medication, posting signs out front saying "we don't carry OxyContin," the Sacklers likely sat back and smiled. Court evidence is unequivocal that illicit use and mass-diversion into the streets was always a part of the firm's plan for *blockbuster* growth in revenue.[59] Referring to Purdue's first patented version of OxyContin, former Rochester County, New York forensic toxicologist James Wesley, speaking to a healthcare industry crowd at a convention in Portland, Maine in 2015, remarked that the formulation of the pills rendered it a ready street drug. Completely pure, the original OxyContin tablets were ready to crush, snort or shoot. There are dozens of available and cheap technologies for making a narcotic pill tamper-proof, and with the original OxyContin, Purdue chose to use

55. John E. Sarno, *The Mindbody Prescription: Healing the Body, Healing the Pain* (New York: Warner Books, Inc., 1999); Gabor Maté, *When the Body Says No: Understanding the Stress-Disease Connection* (Hoboken: Wiley, 2011).

56. The Sackler family was ordered to sell Mundipharma as part of the bankruptcy settlement still being litigated as of the June 2024 US Supreme Court decision to invalidate the deal. The consumer health division of Mundipharma was sold to Singapore-based iNova Pharmaceuticals in January 2024.

57. Kane Wu and Roxanne Liu, "Drugmaker Mundipharma restarts China unit sale in over $1 bln deal – sources," *Reuters*, January 31, 2024, https://www.reuters.com/markets/deals/drugmaker-mundipharma-restarts-china-unit-sale-over-1-bln-deal-sources-2024-01-31/.

58. Future ft. Lil Wayne, "Oxy," track 6 on *WRLD on Drugs*, produced by Richie Souf, Epic, 2018.

59. *Commonwealth of Massachusetts v. Purdue Pharma, L.P.*; Lurie, "'Behave More Sexually.'"

none of them.[60] Court documents unveiled in 2017 from the 2006 federal prosecution of Purdue for willingly misleading the public about the drug's likelihood of abuse, indicate "the company's sales representatives used the words "street value," "crush," or "snort" in 117 internal notes recording their visits to doctors or other medical professionals from 1997 through 1999."[61]

Black market capitalists also deploy brand recognition as an advertising and growth strategy. "Decks" of heroin are branded by the batch, given names that evoke either death or another form of transcendence, meant to convey potency, which equates to desirability, bang for the buck. Decks have names like "Undertaker," "Widowmaker," "Toe Tag," or my personal favorite, seen in Bushwick, Brooklyn in 2017, "Obamacare." Harm reduction groups and peer support networks spread the word on which batches are taking people out or which seemed to leave mysterious, yellow, gummy residue (benzos or another contaminant) in the mixing tin of someone hauled away to the hospital or morgue. Community safety bulletins alert folks for which batch, brand names, to watch out for. But of course, this too doubles as advertising, because when you say, "this is the deck taking people out," what a habituated and seasoned consumer hears is *better, cheaper, faster.* The allure of commodity fetishism's promise is the promise of life in capital's image.

NOT A "WHITE" CRISIS

Misconceptions that characterize the present-day opioid crisis as a "white crisis," both erase the considerable impact of the crisis in non-white communities and obscure the considerably more significant shifting social formations afoot in the twilight of American neoliberalism. The opioid crisis is one vantage from which to understand the shifting contours of racial and national myths of meaning-making.

60.   James Wesley, "The Heroin Narcotic Rx Crisis," presentation at the Northeast Laboratory Association Annual Conference, Portland, Maine, October 22, 2015.

61.   Barry Meier, "Origins of an Epidemic: Purdue Pharma Knew Its Opioids Were Widely Abused," *New York Times*, May 29, 2018, sec. Health, https://www.nytimes.com/2018/05/29/health/purdue-opioids-OxyContin.html.

Whiteness itself is an abstraction born of violence.[62] The rupturing of this once-stable category, along class lines—into categories of upwardly mobile and stuck-in-place (dare I provoke: "globalist" and "deplorable")—is an underexplored contradiction of the present polit-ical-ideological interregnum. White privilege and white supremacy remain dominant material and discursive forces amidst the simul- .
taneous structural production of heightened rates of white peoples' premature death and criminal justice involvement.[63] The contradic-tions belie a plain truth: supremacy hurts everyone. Whiteness by design obscures potential fronts of solidarity, contorts our capacity to see common ground to stand, rewards the beneficiaries with a second serving of the system's slop at the expense of something desirable: being human together.

Princeton economist Angus Deaton, who won the 2015 Nobel Prize for research linking detailed consumption data to aggregate modeling on welfare, poverty, and wealth distribution, published an attention-grabbing study in the same year (co-authored by his wife and fellow Princeton economist, Anne Case) in *The Proceedings of the National Academy of the Sciences* called, "Rising Morbidity and Mor-tality in Midlife among White Non-Hispanic Americans in the 21st Century." The paper surmises quantitative research the pair under-took to investigate the causal linkages behind the "marked increase" in mid-life mortality rates among white Americans between 1999 and 2013. Shorthanded as the "white mortality paper," Case and Deaton found that suicide and drug poisonings were the leading causes driv-ing the new trend in mid-life morbidity and include a discussion of some "potential economic causes."

Case and Deaton also found that mortality rates of white people with no more than a high school degree, which were around 30 per-cent lower than mortality rates of Black people in 1999, grew to be 30

---

62. W. E. B. Du Bois, *Black Reconstruction in America: 1860–1880* (New York: The Free Press, 1998); Martin Bernal, *Black Athena: The Afroasiatic Roots of Classical Civilization* (New Brunswick: Rutgers University Press, 1987); David Roediger, *The Wages of Whiteness: Race and the Making of the American Working Class* (London: Verso, 2007).
63. Anne Case and Angus Deaton, "Rising Morbidity and Mortality in Midlife among White Non-Hispanic Americans in the 21st Century," *Proceedings of the National Academy of Sciences of the United States of America* 112, no. 49 (December 8, 2015): 15078–15083; Vera Institute of Justice, "Overdose Deaths and Jail Incarceration – National Trends and Racial Disparities," 2019, https://www.vera.org/publications/overdose-deaths-and-jail-incarceration/national-trends-and-racial-disparities.

percent higher than Black people by 2015.[64] CDC data corroborates this trend in rising mortality rates for white people in the prime of life (CDC November 2018). "The CDC blamed the increase in drug overdose deaths, as well as a continuing increase in suicides, for a drop in life expectancy in 2017, making that year the third in a row in which life expectancy fell or remained flat."[65]

Data indicate a particularly sharply rising rate of premature death among middle-aged, white American women. Reporting from CDC data, the *Washington Post* called the rate of increase "staggering" and note that drug overdoses, suicides, and excessive drinking are largely accountable for the trend.[66] Analyzing CDC data, another report in the series from the *Washington Post*, titled "A New Divide in American Death," revealed that death rates for white women in their thirties and forties in the US was up 20 percent since 1990, while the death rate for Black and Hispanic women declined slightly in the same period.[67] In the article titled, "White Women Are Dying Faster All Over America—But What About Where You Live?" (2016) the authors highlight the case of Lee County, Virginia, where the death rate for middle-aged white women increased 54 percent since 1999. While the article does not mention Purdue Pharma or OxyContin, Lee County is in the heart of former coal country; it was the first roll-out site for the OxyContin sales campaign and the site of the country's first lawsuit against Purdue.[68]

---

64. Case and Deaton, "Rising Morbidity and Mortality in Midlife among White Non-Hispanic Americans in the 21st Century"; Olga Khazan, "Middle-Aged White Americans Are Dying of Despair," *The Atlantic*, November 4, 2015, https:// www.theatlantic.com/health/archive/2015/11/boomers-deaths-pnas/413971/; Olga Khazan, "Why Are So Many Middle-Aged White Americans Dying?," *The Atlantic*, January 29, 2016, https://www.theatlantic.com/health/archive/2016/01/middle-aged-white-americans-left-behind-and-dying-early/433863/.

65. German Lopez, "She Spent More than $110,000 on Drug Rehab. Her Son Still Died," *Vox*, September 3, 2019, https://www.vox.com/policy-and-politics/2019/9/3/20750587/ rehab-drug-addiction-treatment-sean-blake-opioid-epidemic.

66. Joel Achenbach, Dan Keating, "A New Divide in American Death," *Washington Post*, April 10, 2016, https://www.washingtonpost.com/sf/national/2016/04/10/ a-new-divide-in-american-death/.

67. Joel Achenbach, "'There's Something Terribly Wrong': Americans Are Dying Young at Alarming Rates," *Washington Post*, November 27, 2019, https://www.washingtonpost. com/health/theres-something-terribly-wrong-americans-are-dying-young-at-alarming-rates/2019/11/25/d88b28ec-0d6a-11ea-8397-a955cd542d00_story.html.

68. Van Zee, "The Promotion and Marketing of OxyContin."

Many people are erased in the often-uttered notion that the present-day crisis is a "white people's" crisis.[69] All kinds of people are using opioids and dying from prescription and street-supplied opioids and opiates at markedly higher rates than any time since the American Civil War. A report on the racial and demographic composite of opioid- and opiate-related deaths by the Kaiser Foundation in 2017 found that overdose death rates for Black Americans continued to climb even as late-breaking municipal action (namely naloxone access) began to curb the white death rate.[70] More than five Native American tribes are among the multiparty litigation (what used to be 'class action' lawsuits) against Purdue Pharma.[71] In the last few years, overdose death rates for Black, Hispanic and Native Americans have risen higher than for white people. The Centers for Disease Control and Prevention (CDC) reported that from 2019 to 2020, the largest percentage increase in overdose death rates was observed among Black and Hispanic people. Black Americans saw a 44 percent increase, and Hispanic Americans saw a 40 percent increase, compared to a 22 percent increase among white Americans.

During the first phases of the crisis, when overdose deaths were directly related to pills or the first wave of heroin overdoses as pill prescription clampdowns began, there was a strong demographic over-representation of white and middle-income people. The CDC reported in 2015 that, relative to previous epidemics of drug dependence, large numbers of those affected by opioid and heroin dependence at that

69.   Abdullah Shihipar, "Opinion | The Opioid Crisis Isn't White," *New York Times*, February 27, 2019, sec. Opinion, https://www.nytimes.com/2019/02/26/opinion/opioid-crisis-drug-users.html.

70.   Kaiser Foundation, "Opioid Overdose Deaths by Race/Ethnicity," 2022, https://www.kff.org/other/state-indicator/opioid-overdose-deaths-by-raceethnicity/?currentTimeframe=0&sortModel=%7B%22colId%22:%22Location%22,%22sort%22:%22asc%22%2D%7D.

71.   Stacy L. Leeds, "Beyond an Emergency Declaration: Tribal Governments and the Opioid Crisis," *University of Kansas Law Review* 67, no. 5 (2019): 1013; Committee on Indian Affairs United States Senate, "Opioids in Indian Country: Beyond the Crisis to Healing the Community," March 14, 2018; Sari Horwitz, "3 S.D. Indian Tribes Sue Drugmakers over Opioid Addiction," *Washington Post*, January 10, 2018, https://www.washingtonpost.com/world/national-security/3-sd-indian-tribes-sue-drugmakers-over-opioid-addiction/2018/01/09/7bb50438-f568-11e7-a9e3-ab18ce41436a_story.html.

time were white, middle-income, and possessed of private health insurance.[72]

When licit or illicit supplies of prescription opioids started becoming scarcer, around the time of the 2013 reformulation of OxyContin and the introduction of prescription-monitoring programs and state clampdowns on prescribing practices, white users—having been insulated to a degree from earlier heroin epidemics—were more open to replacing pills with heroin than people from communities with a living memory of the 1970s scourge. While Purdue did its best to fraudulently—criminally, according to Virginia Judge James P. Jones' 2007 verdict—market OxyContin as "nonaddictive," physician racial bias contributed to far lower rates of prescribing to nonwhite patients.[73] The racist state strategy of linking perceptions of heroin use with Black and Brown people as part of a confessed explicit strategy to criminalize liberation movements, coupled with medical industry and physician racial bias against empathizing with Black and Latino patients in pain, contributed to far greater willingness among physicians to prescribe narcotic pain killers to white patients.[74]

A study in California that used geographically specific, race/ethnicity-income quintiles to examine physician prescribing data found startling rates of difference:

> A nearly 300% difference in opioid prescription prevalence across the race/ethnicity-income gradient was observed in California, with 44.2% of adults in the quintile of ZCTAs with the *lowest-income/highest proportion-white population* receiving at least 1 opioid prescription each year compared with 16.1% in the quintile with the highest-income/lowest proportion-white population and 23.6% of all individuals 15 years or older.[75]

---

72. Holly Hedegaard, Margaret Warner, and Arialdi M. Miniño, National Center for Health Statistics (NCHS), "Drug Overdose Deaths in the United States, 1999–2015," *NCHS Data Brief* 274, February 2017, https://www.cdc.gov/nchs/products/databriefs/db273.htm.

73. Barry Meier, "Origins of an Epidemic: Purdue Pharma Knew Its Opioids Were Widely Abused," *New York Times*, May 29, 2018, sec. Health, https://www.nytimes.com/2018/05/29/health/purdue-opioids-OxyContin.html.

74. Dan Baum, "Legalize It All: How to Win the War on Drugs," *Harper's Magazine*, April 2016, https://harpers.org/archive/2016/04/legalize-it-all/.

75. Joseph Friedman et al., "Assessment of Racial/Ethnic and Income Disparities in the Prescription of Opioids and Other Controlled Medications in California," *JAMA Internal Medicine* 179, no. 4 (April 1, 2019): 469–476. Emphasis added.

Disparities in access to medical care, health insurance (private, Medicaid, or Social Security disability), and prescription coverage also contributed to the disproportionate degree to which white Americans were prescribed opioids. Summarizing the findings: low-income, white people were significantly overrepresented in the total population of those receiving prescriptions for opioids.

Racial bias bears on the contours of illicit supply chain distribution of opioids and opiates as well. In *Dreamland*, Sam Quinones documents the extent to which Mexican black-tar heroin supply routes also perpetuated the racial consumption gap in the opioid crisis.[76] Anti-Black racial bias among young Mexican traffickers, as well as fear of encroaching on existing, organized, and defended heroin-selling markets in major cities contributed to Mexican syndicates' penetration of new markets, places where prescription pills first created demand for opioids. Additionally, Quinones reports on the ubiquitous tactic of Mexican startups using white, female heroin-using accomplices (usually encountered outside methadone clinics or Narcotics Anonymous meetings) to introduce the dealers to new markets. These factors further influenced the suburban/rural geographic and white demographic character of the crisis. It's worth noting that Quinones reports that the Mexican sellers who dominated the emerging Midwest and Sunbelt heroin trade were all young men from a single town in formerly agricultural Playa Nayarit, incidentally where ABC films its hit reality series *Bachelor in Paradise*. The young men who travel from Mexico to sell heroin in the US come from communities whose agricultural livelihoods were devastated in the wake of NAFTA. The dislocation theory of addiction, elaborated in Chapter 4, also accounts for supply-side actors' choices among what Karl Marx reminds us are conditions not of one's own choosing.[77]

CHANGING THE KNOWLEDGE BASE
AND ADVERTISING AS EDUCATION

The opioid crisis was not produced by some extraordinary exploitation of "loopholes," but rather is an instance of business as usual in the

---

76. Quinones, *Dreamland*.
77. Karl Marx, *The Eighteenth Brumaire of Louis Bonaparte* (1852), *Marxists Internet Archive*, 2010, https://www.marxists.org/archive/marx/works/download/pdf/18th-Brumaire.pdf.

presently configured institutional arrangements and financial incentives that produce the American healthcare system. The story of Oxy-Contin and its many companion drugs is the story of state capture, wherein compromised and corrupted institutions make policy decisions in an environment without sufficient safeguards protecting the distinction between advertising and knowledge production. Far from a rare case of "regulatory failure," the issue is systemic.

Just like the neoliberal revolution was an ideological campaign sold as sound economic science and enlightened best practice, the so-called "pain management" revolution, for which the foregone treatment was opioid use, was a trumped-up sales pitch masquerading as evidence-based innovation. In the early 1960s, Tennessee senator Estes Kefauver, known for his investigations into the Mafia, chaired a commission on the rapidly growing pharmaceutical industry. His attention was quickly drawn to the Sackler family, and documents summarizing the subcommittee's findings include the following note written by staffers: "The Sackler empire is a completely integrated operation in that it can devise a new drug in its drug development enterprise, have the drug clinically tested and secure favorable reports on the drug from the various hospitals with which they have connections, conceive the advertising approach and prepare the actual advertising copy with which to promote the drug, have the clinical articles as well as advertising copy published in their own medical journals, [and] prepare and plant articles in newspapers and magazines."[78]

Mirroring Arthur Sackler's Valium strategy, Purdue's growth strategy of betting the house on patented opioids came with the launch of a massive, clandestine-but-in-plain-sight, campaign to drum up *awareness*, showcasing new *research*, and sound medical *findings*, about epidemic rates of chronic pain, as well as its own patented formulas for the solution.

In 1999, Tufts University Medical School, in Boston, founded a wholly new master's degree program, the Pain, Research, Education and Policy (PREP) program after receiving a large gift from the Sackler family.[79] An internal university investigation at Tufts found that the

---

78. Keefe, "The Family That Built an Empire of Pain."
79. Joe Walsh and Daniel Nelson, "Inside the Purdue Pharma-Tufts Relationship," *Tufts Daily*, May 19, 2019, sec. Investigative, https://tuftsdaily.com/investigative/2019/05/19/inside-the-purdue-pharma-tufts-relationship/.

relationship with Purdue and the Sacklers compromised the integrity of teaching and research at the medical school.[80] In the 2019 lawsuit, the Massachusetts Attorney General argued that the Tufts-Sackler relationship was a part of the deceptive marketing campaign for Oxy-Contin, an explicit effort to downplay the drug's dangers by partnering with institutions of high repute.[81]

In 2002, a $3 million gift from the Purdue Pharma Fund to Massachusetts General Hospital (MGH) established the "Massachusetts General Hospital Purdue Pharma Pain Center." The director of the new center, Dr. Jane Ballantyne, released a statement: "Too many people today continue to experience pain despite the increasing number of pain relief measures available. This generous gift from Purdue will assist us in finding ways to clear up misconceptions and misunderstandings about pain and provide caregivers with the knowledge and resources they need to help patients who are suffering from pain, perhaps needlessly."[82] The knowledge produced and perpetuated by industry-funded doctors and journals was disseminated by industry funded continuing medical education (CME) courses. Purdue, TEVA, KemPharm, and others provided an in-house, tailored sales pitch modeled to look like cutting edge education to medical professionals (many of whom are required by employers or state licensing boards to earn CME credits annually). This is also not unique to Purdue or to opioid-based drugs, but an industry-wide practice.[83] It is a ubiquitous growth strategy in the neoliberal moment, where actors can be anonymous because dollars are difficult to trace.

80. Allen Frances, "Connecting The Dots Between The Opioid Epidemic And Philanthropy," *Huffington Post*, September 19, 2016, http://www.huffingtonpost.com/allen-frances/connecting-the-dots-between-the-opioid-epidemic-and-philanthropy_b_11996752.html; Andrew Joseph, "How Gifts to Tufts Medical School Advanced Purdue Pharma's Goals," *STAT*, April 9, 2019, https://www.statnews.com/2019/04/09/sackler-purdue-pharma-gifts-to-tufts-advanced-company-interests/.
81. "Commonwealth of Massachusetts v. Purdue Pharma, L.P."
82. Massachusetts General Hospital, "$3 Million Gift from Purdue Pharma to Support MGH Pain Program," 2002, http://www.eurekalert.org/pub_releases/2002-02/mgh-mg020702.php.
83. Michael A. Steinman and Robert B. Baron, "Is Continuing Medical Education a Drug-Promotion Tool?," *Canadian Family Physician* 53, no. 10 (October 2007); "Advertising, Marketing, and Promotional Practices of the Pharmaceutical Industry"; Steven Brill, *America's Bitter Pill: Money, Politics, Backroom Deals, and the Fight to Fix Our Broken Healthcare System* (New York: Random House, 2015).

SHELL GAMES

Cloaked, clandestine actors proliferate in the era of deregulation, and pharma is no exception. The opioid industry funded and supported initiatives that appeared to be grassroots campaigns to influence public opinion and policy regarding access to opioid medications. These initiatives were often designed to downplay the risks of opioid addiction and to advocate for broader access to these medications. The term "astroturfing" refers to fake grassroots campaigns that are actually funded by corporate interests. The opioid industry has been linked to multiple such organizations. Advocacy groups such as the Pain Care Forum, the American Pain Foundation, Pain News Network, the US Pain Foundation, among a host of others, turn up time and again as the sponsors and signatories of a range of self-interested "advocacy" initiatives, co-opting critiques and deflecting unfavorable narratives with legitimate-seeming spin. Recalling Jamie Peck's question about how and why neoliberal policies travel so swiftly across industries and borders, the flood of shell games and half-covered paper trails present a formidable layer of tedium, slogans, intentionally obfuscating noise, rationales, and cynical arguments disorienting even the astute researcher with the sheer mess of it all. AI generated content is quickly compounding this already serious problem. Deregulation and paperwork games allow for an intensification of the departure from the real, by design making it harder to parse advertising from advocacy from evidence.

Patrick Radden Keefe put it plainly in his 2017 exposé on the Sacklers and Purdue: "The marketing of OxyContin relied on an empirical circularity: the company convinced doctors of the drug's safety with literature that had been produced by doctors who were paid, or funded, by the company."[84] Purdue did not act alone in this; it partnered with other opioid-selling firms, like Tel Aviv-based TEVA pharmaceuticals and Endo Pharmaceuticals, among others, all of whom had their own brand-name, patented opioid pills for which they sought the highest possible return on investment.

In December 2011, the American Pain Foundation (APF), which claimed to be "the nation's largest organization for pain patients," was

---

84. Keefe, "The Family That Built an Empire of Pain."

investigated by ProPublica as part of its series "Dollars for Doctors," which examines industry ties to medical knowledge production.[85] ProPublica reported that in 2010, the APF received approximately 90 percent of its $5 million in funding from the pharmaceutical and medical-device industries. The investigation also revealed that the APF's guides for patients, journalists, and policymakers often overstated the benefits and downplayed the risks associated with opioid use.[86] By May 2012, the APF had shut down. [87]

Between 2014 and 2018, several professional associations that had been long-established under the pretense of credible academic and medical science organizations were exposed through congressional research and investigative journalism as being heavily influenced by industry interests. Some of these associations ceased operations, while others continue to function under the guise of legitimate professional organizations. The same issue extends to academic journals that publish research funded by industry, sometimes disguising advertising as scholarly articles.[88]

ROLLOUT

Purdue marketed and launched the drug in places where capitalists had once driven workers hard but has since abandoned them. Using doctor- and place-specific prescribing data from prescription tracking data company IMS Health (now IQVIA) Purdue and its cohort targeted for marketing specific doctors and places where it identified already high rates of opioid pain medicine prescribing, tapping the trend of rising and persistent physical pain among Americans in parts

85. Charles Ornstein, "Pharma Money Reaches Guideline Writers, Patient Groups, Even Doctors on Twitter," *ProPublica*, January 17, 2017, https://www.propublica.org/article/pharma-money-reaches-guideline-writers-patient-groups-doctors-on-twitter.

86. Charles Ornstein and Tracy Weber, "Senate Panel Investigates Drug Companies' Ties to Pain Groups," *Washington Post*, May 8, 2012, sec. Health & Science, https://www.washingtonpost.com/national/health-science/senate-panel-investigates-drug-companies-ties-to-pain-groups/2012/05/08/gIQA2X4qBU_story.html.

87. Ornstein and Weber, "Senate Panel Investigates Drug Companies' Ties to Pain Groups."

88. Matt Kittle, "Who Pays for the Pain? UW's Forgotten Financial Relationship with Purdue Pharma | MacIver Institute," February 11, 2019, https://www.maciverinstitute.com/2019/02/40213/.

of the country where capital had abandoned the working class and left pain in its wake.

Washington County, Maine, for instance, was one of the first places Purdue sent sales representatives. Former logging and paper-mill country, post-industrialization hit northern Maine river and port towns earlier than in other parts of the now enormous American Rust Belt, and the loss of the shoe-making industry in the wake of NAFTA was the final blow. More than one in four working-aged people in Washington County get by on SSDI.[89] The official unemployment rate has in recent decades remained much higher than the state or national average.

Deregulation and "pro-market" policies allowed for lax or no oversight on prescribing, medical records, or pharmacies in most parts of the country. Purdue's sales strategy for OxyContin targeted general practitioners with a focus on what they designated "chronic pain." In a *LA Times* exposé on the firm's replication of this growth and sales strategy in other countries, the investigative journalists write:

> Chronic pain patients, who fill prescriptions month after month and often year upon year, have been the driver of billion-dollar sales for Purdue in the U.S. University of North Carolina researchers analyzed the medical records of patients taking OxyContin at strengths of 30 milligrams or more—common doses for the drug—and found that more than 85% were diagnosed with chronic pain of one type or another."[90]

According to the federal Center for Medicare and Medicaid Services, 42 million Americans receive prescription drug coverage through Medicare Part D. A report released in December 2019 by the American Association of Consultant Pharmacists indicated that Americans in their sixties take *on average* fifteen different prescription medications.[91] The pharma industry, via Medicare and other state subsidies to

89. Michael Stephens, "Disabled-Worker Statistics," June 12, 2018, https://www.ssa.gov/OACT/STATS/dib-g2.html.

90. Harriet Ryan, Lisa Girion, and Scott Glover, "'You Want a Description of Hell?' Oxy-Contin's 12-Hour Problem #InvestigatingOxy," *Los Angeles Times*, May 6, 2016, http://www.latimes.com/projects/OxyContin-part1/.

91. Jane E. Brody, "The Hidden Drug Epidemic Among Older People," *New York Times*, December 16, 2019, sec. Well, https://www.nytimes.com/2019/12/16/well/live/the-hidden-drug-epidemic-among-older-people.html.

private health insurance, amounts to a massive post-Keynesian stimulus program; a systematic transfer of wealth from public coffers to private capitalists.

JUMPING SCALE AND SHIFTING SHAPE

Purdue's strategy to promote "chronic pain awareness" and spread the reckless and dubious gospel of opioid-based chronic pain therapy continues. As OxyContin sales began declining in the United States, around 2010, Purdue began its global strategy, now named as the most significant fact in producing rising rates of opioid dependence and death in other countries.[92] The campaigns use the same tactics—funding biased researchers; partnering with bogus or bought patients' rights groups[93]; and cloaking advocacy as sound medical science in pursuit of the goodwill effort to stop pain.

Mundipharma, Purdue's European division, launched an ambitious OxyContin campaign internationally, and among European countries, particularly focused efforts in Spain. Searching "*dolor*" and "Mundipharma" on Google turns up a whole host of underreported "awareness campaigns" throughout the Spanish-speaking world (and using other languages' word for pain will return similar results for other parts of the world).[94]

One ad from the Spanish campaign, a partnership between el Instituto Mundipharma and la Sociedad Española del Dolor available on YouTube, features nearly nude celebrities. Classic subliminal advertising tactics taught in business school will tell you that shocking material, like nudity, isn't just about getting a viewer's attention for the duration of an ad, but about the synaptic vulnerability to subliminal programming that occurs when a message is delivered in a reasoned and appealing tone alongside imagery that arouses the senses.[95] This ad uses the slogan "*Rebélate contra el dolor*" [Rebel against the pain].

---

92. Alison Branley, "Pharma Giant Hit by Fine for Misleading Local Doctors Over Opioid Drug," *ABC News*, December 23, 2019, https://www.abc.net.au/news/2019-12-23/mundipharma-hit-by-fine-for-misleading-local-doctors-over-opiods/11823280.
93. Lurie, "Behave More Sexually"; Kittle, "Who Pays for the Pain?"
94. Ryan, Girion, and Glover, "'You Want a Description of Hell?'"
95. Joe Dispenza, *Becoming Supernatural: How Common People Are Doing the Uncommon* (Carlesbad, CA: Hay House Publishing, 2017).

Public figures throw off heavy metal chains, defiantly declaring, "This must end!" and "Live!" The ads bundle together back pain, joint aches, hand cramps, and other common conditions to produce a new common-sense notion and a new language of *chronic pain*.[96]

In 2014, a Mundipharma executive stated that since 2007, painkiller sales in Spain were up by 700 percent. In countries where direct-to-consumer advertising prohibitions exist, the firm skirts them with the use of front "advocacy groups." Neoliberalism allowed for this on a global scale. Neoliberalism allowed for the financial deregulation that allowed for shadow partnerships, anonymously funded organizations, shell companies, and other forms of clandestine capital to act in its own and against the public's interest, hiding in plain sight.

The Sacklers played the ubiquitous rebranding game, making the patterns in their insidious tactics difficult to trace as the brand jumps scale and crosses borders. When OxyContin was reformulated in the US in 2011, the firm continued selling the old formula in Canada for years, producing an illicit supply chain of the original, "street drug" formulation into the US from Canada, a route that continues to this day.[97] This has been deemed to be the source of the counterfeit, fentanyl-containing pills implicated in the premature death of beloved artist Prince, as well as countless others.[98]

In 2019 a report released by US House of Representatives members Katherine Clark and Hal Rogers, of Massachusetts and Kentucky respectively, documented the extent to which the knowledge base of the World Health Organization (WHO) had been corrupted by individuals and organizations with hidden ties to Mundipharma, Purdue, and others. WHO guidelines and best practices borrow tactics and phrasing to promote the use of opioid-based treatment as a frontline

96.   Ryan, Girion, and Glover, "'You Want a Description of Hell?'"

97.   "ICES | Canadian OxyContin Prescribing Increased Dramatically near US-Canada Border Following Introduction of Tamper-Resistant Formulation in US: Study," ICES, November 13, 2012, https://www.ices.on.ca/news-releases/canadian-OxyContin-prescribing-increased-dramatically-near-us-canada-border-following-introduction-of-tamper-resistant-formulation-in-us-study/.

98.   "Counterfeit Pills Are Ravaging Communities Across North America," Partnership for Safe Medicines, March 14, 2017, https://www.safemedicines.org/fentanyl-pills-ravaging; "Prince Death: No Criminal Charges to Be Filed," *BBC News*, April 19, 2018, sec. US & Canada, https://www.bbc.com/news/world-us-canada-43829545; Daniella Silva, "Prince Died after Taking Counterfeit Vicodin Laced with Fentanyl, Prosecutor Says," *NBC News*, April 20, 2018, https://www.nbcnews.com/news/us-news/no-criminal-charges-prince-s-overdose-death-prosecutor-announces-n867491.

strategy in the "war against pain." The tactics mirror those used in the previous two decades in the produced American tide change, including significantly downplaying the susceptibility to addiction and naming doctor caution about the drugs "opioidphobia."[99]

REGULATORY ARBITRAGE

In finance as in pharma, "self-regulation" translates to a willful abandonment of the rules in favor of potential profits. Off-label marketing, covert advertising, stacking study panels with 'friendly' and well-compensated experts, buying prestige with endowed chairs and wings and schools of elite institutions—these are all documented strategies undertaken by Purdue Pharma and their opioid-shilling cohort. Business as usual. Pharma's catalogue of legal and illegal improprieties against the public spans a wide array of drug classes and maneuvers. The one commonality is the intention to maximize profits from private and state-funded sales streams, exceed growth targets, and, in the case of publicly traded firms, to raise stock price valuation.

Insurance fraud, and particularly Medicare and Medicaid fraud is another well-documented and explicit growth strategy in the pharmaceutical industry.[100] The firm Insys, currently winding down operations due to bankruptcy stemming from the May 2019 conviction of its founder John Kapoor and four other top executives, were discovered to have defrauded insurance companies in pursuit of growing sales of its patented drug Subsys, a sublingual spray preparation of fentanyl, FDA approved for the treatment of "breakthrough cancer pain." Insys was found to have not only coached doctors' office representatives to lie to insurance companies about a patient's cancer status during pre-authorization checks, often by omitting the word cancer in diagnoses of "breakthrough pain," but also to have run a brazen kickback scheme

---

99. Katherine Clark and Hal Rogers, "Corrupting Influence: Purdue and the WHO," May 22, 2019; Chris McGreal, "Purdue Pharma Accused of 'Corrupting' Who to Boost Global Opioid Sales," *Guardian*, May 22, 2019, sec. US News, https://www.theguardian.com/us-news/2019/may/22/purdue-pharma-opioid-world-health-organization-painkiller-global-sales.
100. Matt Stieb, "Senator Whose Company Defrauded Medicare to Lead GOP's Health-Care Push," *New York Magazine*, April 1, 2019, https://nymag.com/intelligencer/2019/04/rick-scott-is-an-odd-choice-to-lead-gops-health-care-reform.html.

for prescribing doctors. As a perk to doctors prescribing large quantities of the drug, Insys funded the salaries of designated front-office staff, typically the wife or relative of the prescribing doctor, whose sole job was getting insurance approval for patients prescribed the drug, which retailed at between $900 and $3,000 for a thirty-day supply.[101] In a whistleblower lawsuit filed by an Insys sales rep in 2016, the former staff member recalled that when she raised concerns to her supervisors that her imperative to boost Subsys sales might exacerbate the already ongoing opioid epidemic, she was told that Subsys patients were "already addicts and their prospects were therefore essentially rock-bottom."[102] To date, Kapoor is the only pharma executive to serve time in prison relating to criminal involvement in the opioid crisis.

CRIMINAL INTENT

The intention to generate profits from producing mass addiction is clear and irrefutable.[103] From the municipal to the federal and even international scale, the opioid-selling pharma cohort interfered with public safety initiatives, inquiries, and concern whenever and wherever they emerged. Industry consortiums of opioid-selling firms allegedly interfered to quash municipal drug "take back" programs.[104] Lawyers and other hired agents representing industry partners allegedly threatened nurses and doctors who spoke in local press about the dangers of opioid-based chronic pain therapy.[105]

In January 2019, court filings from the Commonwealth of Massachusetts' lawsuit against the Sacklers and Purdue revealed even further evidence of criminal intent that was redacted from earlier cases or newly discovered since then. On January 31, 2019, CNN reported

101. Dina Gusovsky, "The Pain Killer: A Drug Company Putting Profits above Patients," *CNBC*, November 4, 2015, https://www.cnbc.com/2015/11/04/the-deadly-drug-appeal-of-insys-pharmaceuticals.html; Eli Rosenberg, "Maker of Addictive Fentanyl Spray Agrees to Pay $225 Million for Prescriptions-for-Cash Scheme," *Washington Post*, June 6, 2019, https://www.washingtonpost.com/health/2019/06/06/drug-maker-addictive-fentanyl-spray-agrees-pay-million-prescriptions-for-cash-scheme/.
102. Lurie, "Behave More Sexually."
103. *Commonwealth of Massachusetts v. Purdue Pharma, L.P.*; *Lee County v. Purdue Pharma L.P.*
104. Andrew Mannix, "Drugmakers Sue King County over Disposal Program," *Seattle Times*, March 10, 2014, https://www.seattletimes.com/seattle-news/drugmakers-sue-king-county-over-disposal-program/.
105. Quinones, *Dreamland*.

that Sackler family and Purdue lawyers petitioned to keep previously redacted court records concealed that detail family members and high-level employees' "discussions of tactics that could be used to promote the sales of OxyContin (particularly in higher doses), to encourage doctors to prescribe the drug over longer periods of time, and to circumvent safeguards put in place to stop illegal prescriptions."[106] Among the recent disclosures from the Massachusetts case was that the McKinsey Corporation—notorious for its involvement in scandals ranging from Enron to the US Immigration and Customs Enforcement Agency (ICE)—had consulted with Purdue Pharma on tactics for "turbocharging" OxyContin sales.[107]

THE CAPITALIST CLASS CAPTURES THE STATE

In 2007, Purdue and three executives pled guilty to federal criminal charges for misleading regulators, doctors, and patients about OxyContin's risk of addiction and abuse potential.[108] Lee County, Virginia, in former coal country, was an early rollout site and the State of Virginia became one of the first entities to sue Purdue. In 2001, Darrell McGraw, Virginia's attorney general, filed a civil case against Purdue Pharma, alleging that the company used "coercive and deceptive" marketing tactics for OxyContin and that this misinformation campaign led to the drug being prescribed even for minor pain without warning of its highly addictive properties. Purdue recognized the stakes of the case and hired attorney Eric Holder (later US Attorney General under President Obama) of the Washington-based law firm Covington & Burling. In 2004, on the morning of the day a jury trial was set to begin, Holder brokered a deal, settling Virginia's lawsuit for a $10 million payout from Purdue. Purdue executives were not required to admit to any wrongdoing.

---

106. Rob Frehse and Tony Marco, "Opioid Maker Purdue Pharma Fights to Prevent Documents Involving Sackler Family from Going Public," *CNN*, December 1, 2019, https://www.cnn.com/2019/01/30/health/purdue-pharma-stay-bn/index.html.

107. Michael Forsythe and Walt Bogdanich, "McKinsey Advised Purdue Pharma How to 'Turbocharge' Opioid Sales, Lawsuit Says," *New York Times*, February 2, 2019, sec. Business, https://www.nytimes.com/2019/02/01/business/purdue-pharma-mckinsey-OxyContin-opiods.html.

108. Barry Meier, "In Guilty Plea, OxyContin Maker to Pay $600 Million," *New York Times*, May 10, 2007, sec. Business Day, https://www.nytimes.com/2007/05/10/business/11drug-web.html.

Prosecutors in the 2007 federal case against Purdue Pharma and the Sackler family, alongside the Department of Justice investigation, documented that top executives at Purdue were aware early on that OxyContin was being abused. They had knowledge of the drug's involvement in street-use, pharmacy robberies, diversion into illicit markets, and prescription-selling scandals. Despite this awareness, Purdue continued to market OxyContin as having a low potential for addiction. After a thorough four-year investigation, federal prosecutors recommended that three top Purdue executives, including Richard Sackler, be indicted on felony charges, including conspiracy to defraud the United States. However, under the Bush Administration, the case was settled out of court for a substantial fine, avoiding more severe criminal charges.[109]

A dramatically overlooked facet of Purdue's growth strategy, which is not singular to the firm but an industry-wide, profit-seeking tactic, was the flow of revenue from government-funded programs. In fact, firms explicitly build payouts from Medicare and other government sources into their business plan and FDA-approval rationales.[110]

Purdue (among so many other pharma firms), the charge alleged, knowingly made a false claim that OyxContin's patented formulation of generic oxycodone was *worth the cost* to Medicaid, Medicare, Veteran's Administration hospitals, and other state-funded sources of payment for opioids, with the unproven claim that the time-release mechanism eliminated the risk of addiction.[111] With rising numbers of out-of-work, structurally abandoned people in pain getting by on disability checks, Purdue intentionally sought a *state-funded* fix. This exemplifies the degree to which state capture and extraction from state coffers is central to the for-profit medical industry's profit model.

The 2010 Patient Protection and Affordable Care Act, the bundle of legislation that introduced "Obamacare," contained a provision

109. Meier, "In Guilty Plea, OxyContin Maker to Pay $600 Million"; Barry Meier, *Pain Killer: An Empire of Deceit and the Origin of America's Opioid Epidemic* (New York: Random House, 2018); Center for Practical Bioethics, "The IOM Report on Pain," October 26, 2021, https://www.practicalbioethics.org/public-and-population-health/the-iom-report-on-pain/.
110. See, for example, the case of Vivitrol, Suboxone, and the Evzio naloxone auto-injector (discussed in Chapter 7).
111. Soo Youn, "Suboxone Maker Reckitt Benckiser to Pay $1.4 Billion in Largest Opioid Settlement in US History," *ABC News*, July 12, 2019, https://abcnews.go.com/Business/suboxone-maker-reckitt-benckiser-pay-14-billion-largest/story?id=64274260.

requiring the Health and Human Services division to enlist the Institutes of Medicine (IOM) to conduct a national study on the question of chronic pain as a national health problem. The report, which has faced scrutiny for potential pharma lobby influence regarding its findings and recommendations, from among others the Center for Practical Bioethics, was used by the industry as a publicity engine to drum up "awareness" of the pervasiveness of chronic pain. It is alleged that Pharma and industry partners organized to shape the outcome of the study in order to generate a mandate for a national program to address a problem for which they had the fix. The chair of the study, Dr. Philip A. Pizzo, Dean of the Stanford University School of Medicine and a professor of pediatrics, immunology, and microbiology, is prominent in the medical field's discussion of conflict of interest, yet a number of doctors on the study were affiliated with opioid-selling firms and shell advocacy groups.[112] In 2013, when the FDA was criticized for approving patent applications for high-powered, non-tamper-resistant Zohydro-ER, executives evoked the IOM report in their defense, speaking of the need to balance the problem of the opioid epidemic with the mandate of the IOM report to provide meaningful relief to the 116 million Americans suffering from untreated pain.[113]

In 2012, a congressional investigation was launched by the Senate Finance Committee on the connection between opioid sellers and the patients' rights groups and research and advocacy institutions promoting the supposedly safe and effective treatment of pain with opioids, headed by Senators Max Baucus (D-MT) and Chuck Grassley (R-IA). Interest letters asking for funding reports from the Senate committee went to three pharmaceutical companies--Purdue Pharma, Endo Pharmaceuticals, and Johnson & Johnson--as well as five groups that supported pain patients, physicians, or research: the American Pain Foundation, American Academy of Pain Medicine, American Pain Society, Wisconsin Pain & Policy Studies Group, and the Center for Practical Bioethics. Investigators spent months looking into whether

112. Philip A Pizzo, "Oral Presentation to the H.E.L.P. Committee on February 14, 2012," February 14, 2012, 5, https://www.help.senate.gov/imo/media/doc/Pizzo.pdf.
113. Susan Jeffrey, "Attorneys General Ask FDA to Rethink Zohydro ER Approval," Medscape, December 8, 2019, http://www.medscape.com/viewarticle/817702; Pauline Anderson, "Zogenix Files Suit Against State Ban on Zohydro ER," Medscape, April 2014, http://www.medscape.com/viewarticle/823355.

nonprofit medical organizations were receiving money from drug manufacturers to spread misinformation about opioids. Baucus and Grassley left the committee before the release of the investigation, for unknown reasons, and were replaced by Orrin Hatch (R-UT) and Ron Wyden (D-OR), who cut the investigation short and buried the report. Records indicate that Hatch received $177,000 in pain lobby money between 2014–2018.[114] The senators were formally petitioned to release the report in 2015 but kept the document sealed.[115] The next year, Paul D. Thacker, a former investigative reporter for the United States Senate Finance Committee, wrote an article demanding the release of the report, urging Hatch and Wyden to "do your jobs." Speculating on Hatch's motives, not mentioning the lobby money, he suggested his reasons were partly ideological:

> Hatch wants to keep his hands off nonprofits. Why? Hatch holds to an ideological conviction that government is bad and can be replaced by more efficient nonprofits. Releasing a report that hints at how corrupt some of these nonprofits can be would harm that ideology—even as it would help his home state.[116]

In 2018, another report echoing some of the 2012 commission's undisclosed findings was released by the US Senate Homeland Security and Governmental Affairs Committee (HSGAC). It bore the title *Fueling an Epidemic: Exposing the Financial Ties Between Opioid Manufacturers and Third-Party Advocacy Groups*. Published by Senator Claire McCaskill (D-MO), it provided the "first comprehensive snapshot of the financial connections between opioid manufacturers and advocacy groups and professional societies operating in the area of opioids policy."[117] It shows that between 2012 and 2017, a small group of lead-

114. Lenny Bernstein and Scott Higham, "This Company's Drugs Helped Fuel Florida's Opioid Crisis. But the Government Struggled to Hold Them Accountable," *Washington Post*, April 2, 2017, https://www.washingtonpost.com/graphics/investigations/dea-mallinckrodt/.
115. Sabrina Bachai, "The Mysterious Sealed Opioid Report Fuels Speculation," *The Hill*, November 17, 2016, http://thehill.com/blogs/pundits-blog/healthcare/306672-the-mysterious-sealed-opioid-report-fuels-speculation.
116. Paul D. Thacker, "Senators Hatch and Wyden: Do Your Jobs and Release the Sealed Opioids Report," *STAT*, June 27, 2016, https://www.statnews.com/2016/06/27/opioid-addiction-orrin-hatch-ron-wyden/.
117. US Senate Homeland Security & Governmental Affairs Committee (HSGAC), Ranking Member, "Fueling an Epidemic: Exposing the Financial Ties between Opioid Manufacturers and Third Party Advocacy Groups," HSGAC Minority Staff report, https://www.hsgac.senate.

ing opioid manufacturers—among them Purdue Pharma and Janssen Pharmaceutical (subsidiary of Johnson & Johnson)—spent millions on third-party advocacy groups that downplayed addiction risks and endorsed opioid use for the long-term treatment of chronic pain.

There are numerous instances of opioid-dependent firms, pharma companies, distributors, and the sellers of medical pumps and other paraphernalia, intentionally boosting illicit flows of the drugs, turning a blind eye to obvious fraud, pulling favors to quash investigations. Two deserve mentioning for the illumination they offer on the extent to which clandestine class power animates and sets the agenda for governance. In the 2017 Forbes 500 list, which makes note of the rise of healthcare firms into the ranks of the list of the 500 highest-earning US firms, healthcare supply giant the McKesson corporation ranked fifth, behind Walmart, Berkshire Hathaway, Apple, and ExxonMobil. (Fellow health-sector giants UnitedHealth Group and CVS Health come in behind McKesson for sixth and seventh place, respectively.) *Fortune Magazine* reports McKesson's annual revenue that year was $198.5 billion, $4 billion of which came from opioid sales, a decrease from previous years. Their free-flowing taps into pill mills and other black- and grey-market distribution hubs flagged DEA attention in the early 2000s, leading the agency to begin tracking the distribution of pills from McKesson and other firms. Former head of the DEA office responsible for preventing prescription medicine abuse, Joe Rannazzisi, became a whistleblower in 2017, after his agency's years-in-the-making case against opioid pill distributors, including the pharma giant, McKesson, was abruptly halted.

Rannazzisi took over as head of the DEA's Office of Diversion Control in 2006, and the year after, DEA filed an enforcement action against McKesson for failing to report a large number of suspicious orders placed by Internet pharmacies. McKesson settled the case, paying a $13.2 million fine.[118] Rannazzisi recalls being told in 2011 by then-Deputy Attorney General James M. Cole to abandon the case,

---

gov/wp-content/uploads/imo/media/doc/REPORT-Fueling%20an%20Epidemic-Exposing%20
the%20Financial%20Ties%20Between%20Opioid%20Manufacturers%20and%20Third%20
Party%20Advocacy%20Groups.pdf.

118. US Department of Justice, "McKesson Corporation Agrees to Pay More than $13 Million to Settle Claims that it Failed to Report Suspicious Sales of Prescription Medications," May 2, 2008, https://www.justice.gov/archive/opa/pr/2008/May/08-opa-374.html.

but he instead increased the unit's efforts, citing the unit's mandate to prevent drug-related "imminent danger." In the summer of 2014, Rep. Tom Marino (R-PA), drug-czar-to-be under President Trump, proposed a new legislation that would weaken enforcement, changing the previous language to make the bar for legal action much higher. Rannazzisi protested, allegedly saying the new law would protect nefarious actors. In 2016, the bill passed after Sen. Orrin G. Hatch (R-UT) negotiated a final version with the DEA. Between 2014 and 2016, it is reported that the drug industry spent $102 million lobbying Congress on the bill. The twenty-three lawmakers who supported the bill have documented contributions from the industry lobby totaling at least $1.5 million, of which Hatch received $177,000 and Marino close to $100,000. The biggest contributor was the lobby group Pharmaceutical Research and Manufacturers of America (PhRMA), but individual firms also lobbied, including McKesson, with nearly $3 million in contributions. DEA Chief Administrative Law Judge, John J. Mulrooney put the effect of the new law into perspective, saying, it is now "all but logically impossible" for the DEA to suspend a drug company's operations for failing to comply with federal law.[119]

Of course, lobby-funded influence is only part of the story of state capture. The well-known revolving door between government and top corporate firms is another part of the story. Between 2000 and 2017, over fifty ranking DEA and DOJ employees found new jobs in the pharmaceutical industry.[120] In 2004, then retiring Rep. W.J. Tauzin, who had chaired the House Committee on Energy and Commerce, which has shared jurisdiction over Medicare, was recruited to head PhRMA.[121] Tauzin had a key role in drafting and passage of the controversial Medicare Act of 2003 and the inception of Medicare Part D. This industry-written legislation, introducing the infamous "donut hole" scheme, allowed pharma firms to name their price for their drugs, and is hugely responsible for the ballooning drug cost problem that is now another state-funded cash machine for the industry. Bush passed the bill into law in December 2003. On January 3, 2004, the day after he left office, Tauzin started his new job at PhRMA, and in

---

119. Bernstein and Higham, "This Company's Drugs Helped Fuel Florida's Opioid Crisis."
120. Bernstein and Higham, "This Company's Drugs Helped Fuel Florida's Opioid Crisis."
121. Judy Sarasohn, "Tauzin to Head Drug Trade Group," *Washington Post*, December 16, 2004, https://www.washingtonpost.com/wp-dyn/articles/A3504-2004Dec15.html.

2010, he became the highest paid health-law lobbyist in the US, earning $11.6 million.[122]

McKesson settled with the DOJ in May 2017, paying a $150 million fine. The DEA database was released in 2019 following a court order by a US district court judge. *The Washington Post* reported that between 2006 and 2012 (data beyond that is still being withheld "to protect the companies and DOJ investigations"), 76 billion opioid pills were sold, three quarters of which were leading generic formulations, hydrocodone and oxycodone. The top three generic manufacturers, McKesson among them, supplied 87.9 percent of the total pills distributed during the seven-year period, while Purdue Pharma was the fourth biggest supplier, with a 3.3 percent market share. In some counties, such as Mingo County, West Virginia, the numbers were extreme. During the seven-year period, 38,269,630 prescription pain pills were sent there, enough for 203 pills per person in the county, per year. West Virginia in total received shipment of nearly a billion pain pills over this period. Florida, a hotspot for pill mills due to its lax regulations that allowed *prescribing* doctors to also *sell* the pills, received more than 5.5 billion pills.[123]

PAIN'S GAIN

The US division of the Sackler's holdings, Stamford, Connecticut-based Purdue Pharmaceuticals, filed for bankruptcy protection in Fall 2019. It was reported in December 2019 that the family had withdrawn more than $10 billion from the firm in the previous decade, as part of a series of sophisticated accounting maneuvers the family-owned firm is deploying in order to stow away their horde of wealth, to lower the amount that can be seized by the courts in the ongoing multiparty litigation.[124] A bogus settlement offer built on the presumed ongoing sales of OxyContin, which the Sackler lawyers and public relations

122. Alex Wayne and Drew Armstrong, "Tauzin's $11.6 Million Made Him Highest-Paid Health-Law Lobbyist," *Bloomberg*, November 29, 2011, https://www.bloomberg.com/news/articles/2011-11-29/tauzin-s-11-6-million-made-him-highest-paid-health-law-lobbyist.
123. Higham, Rich, and Horwitz, "76 Billion Opioid Pills."
124. Associated Press, "Purdue Payments to Sackler Family Surged after OxyContin Fine," *The Guardian*, December 17, 2019, sec. Society, https://www.theguardian.com/society/2019/dec/17/purdue-payments-to-sackler-family-surged-after-OxyContin-fine.

specialists trumped up to be a $12 billion offer (a figure calculated on the basis of projected *future global sales* in OxyContin) was rejected by more than twenty of the plaintiff municipalities.[125]

The Sacklers became a sensation because we could name them; because, until recently, they wanted their names known and disseminated fractions of their fortune to elite intellectual and cultural institutions. Besides this one notorious family, there remain many unnamed actors playing the same game—with our lives—in the name of extremely high and immediate returns.

Capitalist consciousness' foundational slippage, its departure from the real, was heightened in the neoliberal era, when dollars departed from a metallic base and floating-fiat currencies buttressed financialized, debt-backed regimes of accumulation, an intensification of capitalist violence that hid in discursive and geographical sleights of hand. The neoliberal state apparatus enforced the myth of the benevolence or freeness of the so-called free market while the proliferation of obfuscatory tactics rendered the system's embedded and intensified harms difficult to trace to human actors. These tactics were spatial and cognitive, dislocating capital's crisis articulations as well as *our capacity to perceive them* even as they shaped our daily lives and surroundings. Behind the fourth wall of partitioned capitalist consciousness, the supposed invisible hand colludes in the form of organized class power. The anti-state state works to convert people who do not produce value from labor in the neoliberal regime of outsourced, automated, and degraded labor into conduits through which profits can be realized. This circuitry resolves the problem of effective demand, turning idled, dislocated would-be laborers into a spatial fix, commodity conduits consuming the system's slop, either through private or state-funded means.

Like Wall Street's Big Short in 2008, or the Iraq War, the opioid epidemic was produced as an organized maneuver of dispossession, destruction, and death for profit. Like the 2008 crisis, it remains shrouded in a forcefield of tedious paper trails, rebrands, shell games, and coverups. This is why the project of training our sight,

---

125. Edward Helmore, "'Purdue and the Sacklers Must Be Shut down Completely': Critics Slam Opioids Settlement," *The Guardian*, September 12, 2019, sec. US News, https://www. theguardian.com/us-news/2019/sep/12/opioids-settlement-purdue-sackler-states.

our collective capacity to see capital, must be central to our revolutionary intentions. The capitalist class has been colluding to shape consciousness, producing mass confusion and disorientation alongside mass despair, making the collective unable to see the actors behind the incidents, leaving us with a collective knowing that, as the popular Occupy Wall Street slogan put it, "Shit is Fucked Up and Bullshit." Defeating the regime and collectively creating systems that promote life and thriving necessitates we evolve our collective understanding beyond tautologies and linear, moralistic bad-guy narratives. Training our sight, undoing capitalist consciousness, reintegrating our sense of self, other and the whole, allows for a collective understanding of the nature of the problem from which to begin our conjuring of our collective futures.

The drug economy, licit and illicit, refutes one of the main claims of the discipline of economics: demand drives innovation; "the market steps up to fulfil an unmet need." In fact, capitalism produces supply-side phenomena. Drug epidemics are about new or renewed drugs becoming available as a fix for a fragmented way of life. Capital makes markets through force.

Money in debt-based (fiat) regimes is backed by military might and the state power to turn human beings into money. Addiction and carceral-state circuits of confinement, like debt, spread in regimes of supposed equality, while masking enormous and precipitous rises in inequality of wealth and suffering. The inequality in wealth and suffering produced in pursuit of profit is then tapped as a new revenue stream, churning waste into value and back again.[126] It is this observable circuitry of produced-as-waste-to-recoup-as-value through a named strategy of "rescue" or "improvement" that leads Neil Smith to observe capital's logic of rendering "nature" an accumulation strategy, as well as David Harvey's observation that in the capitalist system, "the body" is also rendered an accumulation strategy.[127]

---

126. Cindi Katz, "Whose Nature, Whose Culture?: Private Productions of Space and the 'Preservation' of Nature," in *Remaking Reality: Nature at the Millenium*, eds. Bruce Braun and Noel Castree, 46–63 (London: Routledge 1998); Vinay Gidwani, "Six Theses on Waste, Value, and Commons," *Social & Cultural Geography* 14, no. 7 (November 1, 2013): 773–783.

127. Neil Smith, "Nature as an Accumulation Strategy," *Socialist Register* 43 (2007): 16–36, https://socialistregister.com/index.php/srv/article/view/5856/2752; David Harvey, "The Body as an Accumulation Strategy," *Environment and Planning D: Society and Space* 16, no. 4 (August 1998): 401–421, https://doi.org/10.1068/d160401.

CHAPTER 4

WHAT OF THE "ADDICT"?

When you call me an 'addict,' you erase everything that is beautiful about me.

—David Zysk, opening remarks, Overdose Awareness March and Vigil, Portland, Maine, August 31, 2015

The question of what transforms a human being into an "addict" gets at the crux of a billion-dollar question on a burning planet: why and by what hidden and plain mechanisms do humans act against our own will and our own best interest? The field of addiction research and medicine is advancing rapidly, and it is not this chapter's aim to reproduce or summarize the scene. The chapter opens with some meditations on addiction that are distilled from research, personal inquiry, and a lifetime of close encounters with, and deep love for, afflicted people. The intention is to push the paradigm shift (of relational, interwoven spacetime) into the center of the room on questions that still too easily slip into a forgotten space of cognitive partition. Even the emerging biopsychosocial model of addiction, addressed later in the chapter, focuses on individuals with a "personal problem."

In this chapter, I seek to weave the so-called "addict" back into the fold of collective, interdependent life by focusing on what the dead but dominant paradigm considers a given—the capitalist world disorder itself. The dominant narratives of the "addict," which shift over time, reveal insights about how the racial, colonial capitalist state maintains legitimacy and reproduces a classed society amid shifting regimes of accumulation.

The chapter ends with some meditations on healing, integration, and recovery. The treatment of addiction in this chapter is intended to create cognitive space in our collective consciousness, to undo the stories of the state and its control regimes. As powerful as any army, as formidable as any jail cell, are the barriers in our own collective understandings of who we are and how life got to be this way. Beyond them lie a new dimension, a *place* we can inhabit, where we can imagine, plan, and choose to enact an entirely new world into being.

DEPENDENCE OR INTERDEPENDENCE

"Addiction" is a complex co-creation between a human being and their environment. It can be summarized as the inability to stop a habit that is pursued in search of relief despite negative consequences inherent to that habit. When we define addiction as "dependency that disintegrates," we can see clearly that addiction is central to capitalism.[1] Capitalism requires and produces dependency that disintegrates and itself is a dependency that disintegrates. The pursuit of compound growth is the cornerstone addiction structuring the dying world's way of life.

An addiction comprises much more than the component parts—substance (material or behavior), person, act of consumption. The perpetual motion of ritualized, habitual comfort-seeking—intention, action, affect, and infrastructure—becomes a reason unto itself. An addiction starts as a conscious choice, a self-soothing strategy, and develops into an entity possessed of its own mind. It is as if something supernatural is involved, like something we can't see enough to understand, let alone change, holds invisible power over us, puppeteers our actions, makes decisions for us. Like capitalism, addictions possess the user, put us under a spell. Like with capitalism, under the illusion of it serving us we come to serve it, even as it eats at the fabric of our existence. We find ourselves acting against our stated intentions and desires for who and how we wish to be. Our choices today have little or nothing to do with our stated goals for the future. We feel alien

---

1. I have adopted this shorthand for addiction from Father Sam Portaro, quoted by Gabor Maté: "The heart of addiction is dependency, excessive dependency, unhealthy dependency—unhealthy in the sense of unwhole, dependency that disintegrates and destroys." See Gabor Maté, *In the Realm of Hungry Ghosts* (Toronto: Vintage Canada, 2018), 131.

to ourselves and isolated from each other. In the absence of a common understanding, we believe another of the system's big lies: there's something wrong with us.

As discussed in Chapter 2, thought-terminating cliches serve empire at the expense of the truth: flawed genes, broken brains, poor choices, demonic dispositions, and disordered desire are commonly recycled and rebranded explanations for the problem of addiction. Whether the problem of the so-called "addict" is ascribed to a moral or medical condition, whether the afflicted is said to be deserving of care or cages, sympathy or stigma, the reigning common-sense conceptions of the so-called "addict" always pivot on logics of individualized disorder. Some people, the story goes, have an irrational, insatiable desire to repeat harmful, self-destructive behavior or consumption patterns. These people are "addicts"; they are not like the rest of us.

"Few other fields of medicine are so powerfully driven by cultural bias and ideology," writes psychiatrist and bioethicist Carl Erik Fisher in his recent book on addiction, *The Urge*. Using one of empire's key narrative devices—*a few bad apples*—the dominant stories of the "addict" seek to contain the critique so as to keep capital on the march. In this way, the slippery and malleable construct of the "addict" does underrecognized and significant service for the legitimacy and maintenance of the state of things.

DISLOCATION AND DEPARTURE FROM THE REAL

Silvia Federici, Walter Rodney, Farida Akhter, and other scholars who help us re-member the world, detail the deliberate effort to erase collective knowledge of our environments, traditions, medicinal plant and faith-based sources of nourishment and sustenance.[2] Focusing on enclosure and capitalist formation in Europe, Africa, and South Asia respectively, all demonstrate that enclosure and the capture of social and natural wealth center on the erasure of knowledge systems and the supplanting of disconnected and dependent ways of being. Karl Polanyi writes in his 1944 work *The Great Transformation*, that the

---

2.   Silvia Federici, *Caliban and the Witch: Women, the Body and Primitive Accumulation* (New York: Autonomedia, 2004); Walter Rodney, *How Europe Underdeveloped Africa* (African Tree Press, 1973); Farida Akhter, "Women and Trees," (Dhaka: UBINIG Publications, 2002).

imposition of capitalism upon peoples and places "must disjoint man's relationships and threaten his natural habitat with annihilation."[3] Polanyi identified this as a central tactic of capitalist development and named it dislocation. Dislocation signifies both removal from the land and the removal of context for people stranded, confined or otherwise left geographically in-place. Drug dependence and the related state of dislocation has a temporal component as well. Dislocation also involves not being able to imagine ourselves in a livable future. Dislocation is the prerequisite destruction of the collective and the commons in pursuit of dependency.

Warfare, fast and slow, is the cornerstone of capital's empire. It is the necessary act that instantiates and maintains exploitative and extractive ways of being. Forced forgetting is central to the project of market, money, and profit-centric social relations. The intention is to extinguish the light of consciousness, the torch that illuminates resistance, rebellion and dissent to the imposition of extractive logics. It happens through instantaneous ruptures, such as in war, or declaring certain languages or faith traditions criminal.[4] More difficult to detect are the ways it happens over slow expanses of time, as forms of what Rob Nixon names "slow violence" and Dean Spade identifies as "administrative violence."[5]

Forced forgetting is a project of erasure and the essence and extent of the hermeneutic violence baked into the present paradigm. It is essential to the creation of knowledge systems based in abstractions and social (dis)orders based on quantification. The production of abstract space is a necessary precursor to a social disorder predicated on abstract wealth. It makes uniformity, order, out of the beautiful mess of life lived in context, in place, on a living Earth. French

---

3. Karl Polanyi, *The Great Transformation: The Political and Economic Origins of Our Time* (Boston: Beacon Press, 2001), 42.
4. My time living in Bangladesh and becoming friends and kin to veterans of the Bangla language movement (ভাষা আন্দোলন or *Bhasha Andolôn*) and the Liberation War taught me a lot about recognizing these patterns. My time living in Argentina and becoming a student of the movement for the remembrance of *Los Desaparecidos* [The Disappeared], taught me a lot about recognizing these patterns. Studying my ancestry, my grandmother's life in British Occupied Ireland and my grandfather's life in the final days of Ottoman Salonica, taught me a lot about recognizing these patterns.
5. Rob Nixon, *Slow Violence and the Environmentalism of the Poor* (Cambridge, MA: Harvard University Press, 2013); Dean Spade, *Normal Life: Administrative Violence, Critical Trans Politics, and the Limits of Law* (Brooklyn: South End Press, 2011).

philosopher Henri Lefebvre remarked that abstract space, a production of violence, "serves those forces which make a tabula rasa of whatever stands in their way, of whatever threatens them—in short, of differences."[6] Forced forgetting produces the necessary prerequisite for seeing the way the current world disorder needs us to see. It goes hand and hand with another process I call the *departure from the real*, the project whereby new ways of seeing and knowing, the fractured stories needed to sell a collective consciousness conducive the maintenance of a power-over, extractive social disorder are imposed. These knowledge systems promote the collective passive consent to participation in a harm-based economic system that is against life itself. Stripping context from people, life and place produces disorder. It is the absence of this very context that then allows for the critical misdiagnosis, the inversion of reality wherein people made unwell by a sick way of life get labeled "disordered."

COMMODITY COMFORT AND THE QUEST FOR RELIEF

The history of the modern world can be told through the lens of commodities. In *The Making of the English Working Class* (1966), E.P. Thompson discusses the important tactical role of Indian-grown tea.[7] Sydney Mintz tracks the importance of the adoption of sugar in global working class and elite consumption patterns in *Sweetness and Power* (1986).[8] Thompson describes sweet, strong tea as a cheap stimulant and caloric provision in industrializing Britain; how the substance supplanted the need for workers to take time away from value-producing labor for the nonproductive acts of eating and resting. In being a cheap source of calories and energy, heavy consumption of sugary tea allowed for the cost of short-term reproduction of the workforce to remain low enough to keep wage rates suppressed.

The story of the making of the present-day American opioid crisis follows an observable and well-worn pattern in the history of

---

6.   Henri Lefebvre, *The Production of Space*, trans. Donald Nicholson-Smith (Malden: Wiley-Blackwell, 1992), 285.

7.   E. P. Thompson, *The Making of the English Working Class* (New York: Vintage, 1966).

8.   Sidney Wilfred Mintz, *Sweetness and Power: The Place of Sugar in Modern History* (New York: Penguin Books, 1986).

capitalism of the concerted effort not to meet market demand but to manufacture a market for a given commodity. A commodity is a good produced uniformly and en masse and sold on a market. The allure of a commodity is that it appears as if from nowhere and no one. The labor, inputs, and production processes are invisibilized by design in capitalist commodity-centric consciousness.

Alienation is the primary affective state of life under capitalism. Alienation occurs, as Marx catalogued it, from the product of our labor, our labor process, from our human potential, and from one another. This fundamental severing is essential to maintaining the disorder of things. True belonging and satisfaction go against the system's existential need to produce division and unmet needs—and thus a cheap labor force—as well as insecurity and fear, which are the backbone of the imperialist state's power regime. In lieu of satisfying our true needs, the commodity-centric world disorder presents us with a dazzling array of items for sale, none of which satisfy what we really need or truly want.

Comfort-seeking through commodity consumption is endemic in the capitalist mode of production. Advertising ensures that an affective linkage between comfort and consumption are programmed into the populace. The system in fact, turns us all into addicts. We consume because it is what is on offer to correct for a pervasive sense of being out of balance, off center, seeking two essential elements of life that by design must remain out of reach in the dead paradigm: meaning and belonging.

"GOD, SCIENCE, OR SOME AMALGAM OF THE TWO"

Scientism—adherence to the Western scientific method—and the medical model born from it are wedded to the dead but dominant paradigm's partitioned frame. In the case of so-called addiction and the medicalization of "substance use disorder," medical models seek to contain the narrative of mass suffering and disordered consumption by locating the problem in supposedly disordered human beings, either in genes or "diseased brains." Scientific, abstracted modes of explanation have long been central strategic tools of imperial power.

Determinism is a crucial component of the thought paradigm and reductive logics of imperial science.

As Richard Peet notes, historically "determinism attempted to explain the imperial events of late nineteenth and early twentieth century capitalism in a scientific way."[9] Regarding the strategic utility of this approach for the ruling classes (and the geographers who sought their favor and employment), Peet elaborates, "The need to escape from guilt over the destruction of other peoples' lives, a guilt that survived even in a racialist view of the world, meant that the motivations for actions had to be located in forces beyond human control—'God,' 'Nature,' or some amalgam of the two."[10]

Determinism forecloses our understanding of how things come to be, and pessimism forecloses our capacity to imagine what could be otherwise. The history of thought and official policy toward the "addict" is rife with both. Biologically deterministic explanations of addiction are common. A chapter in the official "Big Book" from Alcoholics Anonymous, titled "The Doctor's Opinion," hypothesizes that alcoholism results from a physical allergy to alcohol.[11] Biological explanations for so-called addiction focus on theories of faulty brain functioning and sometimes seek genetic causality.[12] The National Institute on Drug Addiction (NIDA)'s long-term promotion and support of the "brain disease" model has been characterized as an effort to bring "a unified framework to a problem-based field in conceptual disarray.[13] The brain disease framework rests on a theory of malfunctioning neurotransmitters in the reward centers of the brain, which may be genetically predisposed. Embedded in the theory is the corresponding belief in a pharmacological cure. The "brain disease model of addiction" has

---

9. Richard Peet, "The Social Origins of Environmental Determinism," *Annals of the Association of American Geographers* 75, no. 3 (1985): 309–333.

10. Peet, "The Social Origins of Environmental Determinism."

11. Alcoholics Anonymous World Services. *Alcoholics Anonymous: The Story of How Many Thousands of Men and Women Have Recovered from Alcoholism.* 4th ed. New York: Alcoholics Anonymous World Services, 2001.

12. P. W. Kalivas, N. Volkow, and J. Seamans, "Unmanageable Motivation in Addiction: A Pathology in Prefrontal-Accumbens Glutamate Transmission," *Neuron* 45, no. 5 (March 3, 2005): 647–650; Francesca Ducci and David Goldman, "The Genetic Basis of Addictive Disorders," *The Psychiatric Clinics of North America* 35, no. 2 (June 2012): 495–519.

13. Nancy D. Campbell, *Discovering Addiction: The Science and Politics of Substance Abuse Research* (Ann Arbor: University of Michigan Press, 2007); Rachel R. Hammer et al., "The Experience of Addiction as Told by the Addicted: Incorporating Biological Understandings into Self-Story," *Culture, Medicine and Psychiatry* 36, no. 4 (December 2012): 712–734.

dominated research agendas and federal research funding priorities on 'addiction' since the mid-nineties. NIDA, which supports more than 85 percent of the world's research on "drug abuse" and "addiction," is governed by leadership that favors the brain-disease model. Other dominant agencies also lend credence to the biological mode. The American Society of Addiction Medicine has defined addiction as a "primary, chronic disease of brain reward, motivation, memory, and related circuitry."[14]

The genetic, brain-disease and biological determinist models of addiction are appealing for the simplicity of cause begets effect. This gives human animals a sense of control. The dead but dominant paradigm loves control.

Determinism signifies an oversimplification and linear thinking in reductive, causal explanation. As divine-rights logics lost sway to scientific ideas coincidental with liberal, pro-market social order—what some call the "Kantian turn"—deterministic explanations, rooted in geographical, biological, or other supposedly natural causes offered 'rational' justification for imperial conquest and domination.[15] Geographer James Blaut summarized the ideological origins of determinism, saying, "most European intellectuals took it for granted that a Christian god would favor his own people, Christian Europeans, providing them with racial, cultural, and environmental superiority over all others. . . . Later, overtly religious explanations became unpopular, and Europe's (or the West's) superiority was attributed mainly to race and environment, held jointly to have created a uniquely progressive culture."[16]

While racial modes of explanation eventually lost sway in scientific explanation in the shifting ideological order of what Jodi Melamed calls "racial liberalism," environmentalist modes of explanation persist in popular culture, development, and environmental policy research and throughout the physical and social sciences.[17] Blaut notes

14. American Society of Addiction Medicine General Information Flyer, c. 2017, https://www.asam.org/docs/default-source/advocacy/2-asam-general-information-flyer.pdf?sfvrsn=3c6f46c2_2.

15. Livingstone, The Geographical Tradition, 113.

16. James M. Blaut, "Environmentalism and Eurocentrism," Geographical Review 89, no. 3 (1999): 391–408.

17. Jodi Melamed, Represent and Destroy: Rationalizing Violence in the New Racial Capitalism (Minneapolis: University of Minnesota Press, 2011).

the appeal of determinism, in particular how the seemingly neutral and scientific category of the "environment" appears to offer concise answers to complex questions.

Gabor Maté states the dialectical truth purposefully omitted in the individualistic, determinist mode: "The part that Buddha didn't say is that before our minds create the world, the world creates our minds."[18] A dialectical framing centers the conditions under which "disordered" brains come into being. Rather than genetics or biology, the best research on the question locates the root causes of the problem of so-called addiction in childhood trauma and pervasive (occurring or potentially present) threats to survival experienced by human beings in early childhood, when the brain is developing. Exposure to traumatic stress, particularly early in life, is a major factor in the production of the propensity for developing an addiction. The reasons for this are complex, partly having to do with the way a brain and nervous system exposed to traumatic experiences (including abandonment, neglect, and chronic instability in childhood) develop, partly to do with the ways alienation and self-worth are unevenly distributed, partly to do with personality structure, and some part genetic inheritance or biological wiring. The imperialist science paradigm is partial to the latter factors because, as with everything the paradigm favors, it can be spliced, diced, isolated, quantified, and studied in abstraction.

Recent years has seen the rise of a relational, contextual understanding of the phenomenon, the biopsychosocial model of addiction. This framework blends emotional, biological, social, and environmental factors into its understanding of the condition and proposed policy responses and is beginning to crack the veneer of the old paradigm of partition. The dead but dominant paradigm still rules the public imaginary and animates the state-sponsored response efforts on the condition. These perspectives vary depending on time, place, and context but paint the problem of addiction as an anomaly and an individual rather than social problem. While the biopsychosocial model is a relational theory and thus an improvement in leaps and bounds over the moral/medical, individual-pathology model of so-called addiction,

---

18. Gabor Maté and Sat Dharam Kaur, "Compassionate Inquiry Training Material," *Dr. Gabor Maté*, December 20, 2018, https://drgabormate.com/announcing-the-compassionate-inquiry-online-training/.

it still frames the problem as something to fix within the current world disorder. Decolonizing means divesting from the fetish of quant-driven techno-fixes. It's the paradigm that needs changing.

HOW A CLASS SOCIETY IS MADE AND MAINTAINED

Socially and structurally devalued categories of human beings are not only useful but necessary in capitalism. The notion of "the addict" helps us see how capitalism survives by externalizing and individualizing its essential nature as a dependency that deteriorates. Outsourcing and off-shoring the collective shadow onto groups of people who are positioned to absorb social blame is a key strategy of the ideological apparatus of empire and the capitalist state. It is a central strategy in the production, reconfiguration, and reinforcement of a classed society. The story of the so-called addict, an individual with disordered consumption, wipes away the sins and the embedded social dysfunction of a global economic system structured on insatiable ways of being. Ignoring the historical, social, and structural contexts that produce people in need of commodity-based coping mechanisms diverts attention from the capitalist system itself and onto supposedly flawed (groups of) individuals. As with every other systemic problem under capitalism, enormous human potential and collective problem-solving effort (in earnest, as well as the dominant attempt to cover-up and co-opt the critique with rebranding and window dressing) then goes in to trying to remedy a discrete manifestation of capitalism's systemic social and ecological harm. In the absence of collective capacity see the interrelatedness of profit and pain, growth and *golpe*, we divert resources and lifeforce into trying to reverse engineer, regulate, or otherwise ameliorate the system's embedded, perpetual, and perpetually worsening harm.

It is a generalizable trait of the racial capitalist state's method of control, what Ruth Wilson Gilmore names the "individualization of social disorder."[19] Individualization is a strategy for externalizing

---

19. Ruth Wilson Gilmore, *Golden Gulag: Prisons, Surplus, Crisis, and Opposition in Globalizing California* (Oakland: University of California Press, 2007); Ruth Wilson Gilmore, "Race, Prisons and War: Scenes from the History of US Violence," *Socialist Register* 45, no. 45 (March 19, 2009), http://socialistregister.com/index.php/srv/article/view/5897.

endemic, produced, and preventable harm. Throughout its shifting formations, capital's agents and attendant state apparatuses keep the system afloat by discursively, cognitively, ideologically, and spatially externalizing the human beings upon whom its inherent violence is thrust, thereby securing the passive consent of the masses. It partitions the population into a constantly mutating "us-versus-them" in attendant economic regimes of accumulation and control. It is in this way the biopsychosocial model—the most humane, research-based, and socially sound approach to treating the problem of individuals with dependency issues—is still destined to fall short of being a real solution. Prevention-focused efforts seek to address the capitalist system's embedded propensity for drug-based coping mechanisms but not alienation—dislocation from self, other, and collective contexts—and its key role in the "addiction supply industry."

IDEOLOGY, PARTITION, AND "THE ADDICT"

Governance regimes in racial, colonial capitalism spin stories meant to justify who gets cake and who gets cages—or in the present-day case of "the addict," who gets cages and who gets equine therapy. Tracking how the concept of "addiction" and the specter of "the addict" moves in public discourse and policy helps us to see how racialism—the partitioning of human beings into group-differentiated hierarchies of goodness, deservingness, and humanity—is a central feature of capitalism's and empire's governance regime. *Charity and sympathy* and *blame and punishment* are imperialist crisis containment strategies involving the production and reconfiguration of class-based partitions in belonging and exclusion. Examining the shifts between *sympathy and stigma*—alongside shifting regimes of economic accumulation and their attendant regimes of racial order—reveals the nature of the racial, caste, and other kinds of hierarchical partitioning tactics, technologies of domination that stoke within the populace a perception of supposedly natural or just divisions.

The history of how the dominant ideology and science of the disordered paradigm has sought to explain, rationalize, pathologies, stigmatize, control, remove, or resolve the problem of addiction illustrates the main containment strategies in the toolbox of racial, colonial capitalism. The shapeshifting explanatory framework for the condition of deleterious dependency offers a vantage on the dead but dominant paradigm's inherent strategy to pathologize and externalize its rampant internal disorder. Criminalization and medicalization are two sides of the same coin of crisis containment.[20] The strategies overlap and transmute, both operating as what Gilmore teaches as the carceral, racial capitalist state's strategy of individualizing social disorder.[21]

In the dead but dominant framework, stories of the "addict" rest on commodity fetishism, which imbue the substances themselves with the power to possess, and deterministic theories of flawed biology and overtly dehumanizing (racist, classist, and shame-based) ideas of moral failure. The personalizing and pathologizing narratives that animate the so-called "addict" in the human drama of epidemics of mass dependency and premature death exist on a continuum of moral to medical modes of explanation, exhibiting a central fulcrum of imperialist ideology. In examining trends in the development of the concept, common sense and consensus for appropriate response to the condition of addiction and to outbreaks of epidemics of substance-use-related premature death, we approach the dominant paradigm from a different angle. We examine some produced but taken-for-granted assumptions about the so-called "addict" in a paradigm existentially bound to irrational, deleterious consumption. In doing so, we dislodge a boulder in the collective imaginary. *Consciousness is the coming into awareness that you are colonized,* I repeat as a refrain, the words of my friend and comrade Sónia Vaz Borges.[22]

Estimates suggest the United States spends about five times as much money prosecuting and incarcerating people with substance use disorder as it would cost to treat them. Of the nearly two million people incarcerated in the United States, the National Institute on Drug Abuse (NIDA) estimates that about 65 percent has an active substance use disorder,[23] and many others were incarcerated due to crimes committed as a result of drug use, such as drug trafficking or theft to

20.   Peter Conrad, "Medicalization and Social Control," 24.
21.   Gilmore, *Golden Gulag.*
22.   Sónia Vaz Borges, presented during a seminar in the Center for Place, Culture, and Politics in 2017 and scribbled in my notebook and mind. I first evoked the phrase in Chapter 2.
23.   NIDA, Criminal Justice Drug Facts, https://nida.nih.gov/publications/drugfacts/criminal-justice.

support a drug habit. Additionally, the National Center on Addiction and Substance Abuse at Columbia University had previously reported that over 80 percent of all inmates had a history of substance dependence. Carceral state expansion and criminal-confinement-based solutions to the problem of drug dependence persist even amidst the shifting official conception of the condition as a "disease" or medical condition (see Chapter 7).

CHANGING DISCOURSE

Capitalism thrives on split consciousness, suppressed emotions, and inhumane ways of being. Like other contradictions that threaten the status quo, the power structure responds to new outbreaks of epidemic suffering or humanitarian crisis when it must. Like all extractive institutions, the state prefers of course to sweep its problems under the rug. Thus, evolution in the "official story" of the problem of mass dependency occur only in the wake of a rupture that threatens the established order. Official stories about addiction, "addicts," and attendant state-sanctioned response strategies change when the crisis apparent in the problem of epidemic dependence can no longer be managed within the existing ideology. Like with all paradigm shifts, when too much "data" become "outliers" to the existing models, mass dissent, rebellious questioning and critique spur politicians, spin doctors, and salivating profiteers into action—*contain the narrative. Maintain control. Make a buck. Win the polls.*

These official white lies or "bourgeoise historiographies," as Cedric Robinson put it,[24] exploit our mind's preference for simple, neat, and linear narratives. It bears repeating that this bias for simplistic narratives renders us, as a species, vulnerable to explanations that inherit the flattened, reductive moralism that is ultimately friendly to the paradigm.[25] A crucial challenge of the present moment is to clearly

24.   Cedric J. Robinson, "Capitalism, Slavery and Bourgeois Historiography," *History Workshop Journal* 23, no. 1 (March 1987): 122–140, https://doi.org/10.1093/hwj/23.1.122.
25.   I am thinking of the tautological critique levied in, for example, *The New Jim Crow* or the film *The 13th*, as opposed to the revolutionary materialist expositions offered in *Black Reconstruction in America* and *Golden Gulag*. The first coupling dead-end in moralism and pessimism; the second are roadmaps, field guides, weapons.

articulate the dialectical, historical, and present machinations of racial and other technologies of partition.

Jodi Melamed's concept of racial liberalism, articulated in her 2011 book *Represent and Destroy*, critically examines how liberal ideologies, which promote equality and individual rights, have been historically and contemporarily intertwined with the perpetuation of racial inequalities. Melamed identifies "historic repositories and cultural, spatial and signifying systems that stigmatize and depreciate one form of humanity for the purpose of another's health, development, safety, profit or pleasure."[26] Bringing to the fore the use of stigma and sympathy as dialectically related modes of racialism—which is to say, effective for enforcing partitioned social hierarchy—is illuminating in the case of the so-called addict. Melamed's framing, along with other scholars who take a dialectical approach to understanding the contours of race and class in the long arc of capital's empire, offers a framework for thinking through these by-design landmines of what changes and what stays the same amidst capital's machinations to stay in control.[27]

This universal tactic of liberalism recalls the George Harrison song, *Isn't It a Pity?* When my parents' neighbors, coworkers, and friends were losing their homes to foreclosure, their children to overdoses and senseless wars, their pensions to the *golpe growth* machine, I'd often interrupt the mantra, *isn't it a pity*, with "*it's not a pity or a shame. It's criminal.*" I'm also reminded of the famous quote from Utah Phillips, "The earth is not dying, it is being killed, and those who are killing it have names and addresses."

I remember how, during our meetings about my dissertation, David Harvey would encourage me to evidence my hunches about the overlap between foreclosure rates and Oxy prescription and overdose death rates. This was before public consciousness arose about the "deaths of despair" set, the two-time-Obama-turned-Trump-voting set, the dispossessed and disillusioned formerly white working class. Encouraging me to make the case, he'd say, "*It's a 'whodunit?' In the final act, who is holding the gun?*"

---

26. Melamed, *Represent and Destroy*, 152.
27. Cedric Robinson, Paul Gilroy, and Nikhil Singh, among others.

SYMPATHY, STIGMA, AND THE COLOR LINE

Sympathy and stigma are tactics of partition. Sympathy begets charity; stigma begets abandonment or punishment. Both amount to discursive-ontological devices—stories that are productive of ways of seeing—that individuate and pathologize structurally embedded suffering. Historical record shows "addiction" was not thought of as a "condition" nor as a law-and-order societal concern until it involved people of lower classes, who were not of European descent, and whose intoxication was more likely to spill over into public space.[28] The first modern mention of "addicts" and "addiction," rather than describing habitual users and dependency, comes in reference to working and workless poor Chinese immigrants experiencing bad economic luck in the wake of the bust-phase of the California gold rush with its attendant railroad-building and economic boom. Social panic first arose and was mobilized in the name of the spectral figure of "the addict" when unseemly intoxication amidst suffering occurred in public and by nonwhite, non-Western people at a time of economic scarcity. Before this, mentions of dependency on the morphine molecule were treated with sympathy.

During the American Civil War, opium poppies were cultivated in Virginia, South Carolina, and Georgia to produce morphine. Use of morphine among soldiers, for both the acute pain of battle-inflicted wounds, as a remedy for dysentery, and for the prolonged condition of war trauma—then called "shell shock"—led to the existence of thousands of morphine-dependent former soldiers in the aftermath of the war. Metzger says, "The American Civil War did more to create the desire and need for morphine than any other force. More soldiers died in the conflict from diarrheic dysentery than from gunshot wounds. And morphine provided relief for both these conditions."[29] Habituation and continued use of the drug after the acute phase of treatment was widespread and became known as "the soldiers' disease," and former soldiers with morphine dependency were called *habitués*. The

---

28. Th. Metzger, *Birth of Heroin and the Demonization of the Dope Fiend* (Port Townsend, WA: Breakout Productions Inc., 1998); Martin Booth, Opium: A History (New York: St. Martin's Griffin, 1999); Alisse Waterston, *Street Addicts in the Political Economy* (Philadelphia: Temple University Press, 1997); David T. Courtwright, *Dark Paradise* (Cambridge, MA: Harvard University Press, 2009).
29. Metzger, Birth of Heroin, 6.

drug's use spread not only to those directly involved in combat but also became a popular tonic for the grief associated with the loss of life caused by the war. "Maimed and shattered survivors from a hundred battlefields, diseased and disabled soldiers released from hostile prisons, anguished and hopeless wives and mothers made so by the slaughter of those dearest to them, have found, many of them, temporary relief from their suffering in opium," wrote Dr. Horatio Day in his essay, *The Opium Habit* (1868).[30]

The medical/moral dialectic contains two central pivoting conceptions—one is around the legitimacy of use, which ultimately amounts to culturally produced notions of legitimate and illegitimate pain and pain management; the other, more broadly applies to the question of whether addiction is an immoral choice or a biologically conscripted disease. Research on the latter theory centers on the quest to locate a causal determinant, typically either a gene or a mechanically broken brain. Licit and illicit consumption of opioids has historically centered on this bifurcation of legitimate and illegitimate pain and use. The spatial partition of private and public is central to this divide as well, rendering visible the racial containment strategy of drug prohibition logics and legislation.[31] Sympathy and stigma are both tactics of racial partition in shifting regimes of official meaning-making. Exploring habitual drug consumption and so-called disordered use in different historical spacetimes helps to excavate the shapeshifting ideological contours of the eruption and containment of embodied social crises in capital's empire. Freud, whose personal enthusiasm for and habitual use of cocaine is well documented,[32] recognized something like the afterlife of traumatic experience in women patients and named it "hysteria," one of the treatments for which was morphine.

Epidemiological studies of opioid dependence between 1878 and 1885 conducted in Michigan, Iowa, and Chicago determined that more

---

30. Quoted in Metzger, *Birth of Heroin*, 6.
31. Beth Macy, "America's Other Epidemic," *Atlantic*, April 15, 2020, https://www.theatlantic.com/magazine/archive/2020/05/nikki-king-opioid-treatment-program/609085/; Max Mishler, "Race and the First Opium Crisis," *Boston Review*, April 9, 2019, http://bostonreview.net/forum/how-race-made-opioid-crisis/max-mishler-race-and-first-opium-crisis; Alfred McCoy, "The Stimulus of Prohibition: A Critical History of the Global Narcotics Trade," in *Dangerous Harvest*: Drug Plants and the Transformation of Indigenous Landscapes, ed. Michael K. Steinberg et al. (Oxford: Oxford University Press, 2004), 24–111; Booth, *Opium: A History*.
32. Howard Markel, *An Anatomy of Addiction: Sigmund Freud, William Halsted, and the Miracle Drug Cocaine* (New York: Vintage, 2011).

than 60 percent of those dependent on the drug were women from the upper classes in their thirties and forties.[33] Women of European descent, particularly upper-class housewives, had been heavy opium and derivative substance consumers for decades before public outcry over consumption of the drug, as a treatment for hysteria, neurasthenia, and other pathological delineations for the psychosocial-somatic afflictions associated with the captive and dehumanized status of well-off women.[34] Doctors made regular house calls to administer, resupply and renew prescriptions for opium, morphine, and laudanum in the name of treatment.[35]

Opium and its derivatives were the subject of the first international agreements on any substance or commodity in the modern era. In 1906, in part due to the headache of managing an inherited Spanish colonial regime for licensing and providing opium to dependent people in the Philippines, Theodore Roosevelt called for an international conference on opium. The first conference was held in Shanghai in 1909. Two subsequent conventions were held at the Hague in 1911 and 1912, the second of which produced the first international drug control treaty, the International Opium Convention, signed in January 1912 at the Hague. This conference marked the beginnings of international cooperation and discussion over drug control with virtually all major international powers taking part, but it also highlighted a dramatic difference between the US and Europe over their ideological approaches. This divergence in approaches stemmed from opposing views related to drugs and drug dependence. The US supported complete prohibition, viewing addiction as a weakness of character, and saw the drug trade as a dangerous problem that could only be terminated through harsh criminal sanctions and the elimination of supply. Folly of course always lies in prohibition, which amounts, under capitalism, to an unregulated market. Scholars on the drug trade commonly extoll the "stimulus of prohibition,"[36] that banning drugs actually encourages new illicit producers to enter the market, as the potential windfall rises

33. Metzger, *Birth of Heroin*, 9.
34. Nancy Campbell, *Discovering Addiction: The Science and Politics of Substance Abuse Research* (Ann Arbor: University of Michigan Press, 2007), 12.
35. Markel, *An Anatomy of Addiction*, 9.
36. McCoy, The Stimulus of Prohibition; Planet Money, "The Moonshine Stimulus," *NPR*, August 3, 2010, https://www.npr.org/sections/money/2010/08/03/128960709/the-tuesday-podcast.

with the stakes. Europe on the other hand, favored a medical approach, supporting the need for treatment facilities and gradual reduction of drugs. This conflict of interest spawned in part because the United States had no vested interest or economic reliance on the colonial drug trade. Europe, on the other hand, was still heavily invested in the economy of the drug trade, and feared that strict regulation would lead to more illicit criminal activities.[37] This first act of prohibition in the United States, the Harrison Narcotics Act, passed into law in 1914, sought to curtail the non-medical uses of opium and coca products, as a response to public concern over opium addiction and addicts, a racialized panic in the context of economic decline.

Flawed genes, *dirty brains*, poor choices, demonic dispositions, and disordered desire are commonly recycled and rebranded explanations for the problem of so-called addiction, always logics of individualized disorder, always rooted in racist constructs that allow for mass-produced cognitive dissonance from this among many formations of human suffering produced in accordance with social (dis) orders animated by the quest to accumulate power and profit. So-called addiction is a coping and self-soothing strategy, its root cause is traumatic stress, the lived afterlife of violence that is central to capitalism's disordered world.

Racialism is a technology of social partition that predates capitalism but is deployed and renovated by capitalist/state agents in pursuit of growing profits and ongoing legitimacy. Racial logics, the categories and the meanings put to work about them, have "viscosity," according to Arun Saldahna, author of *Psychedelic White* (2007). They are mutable, changing, and yet fixed in the collective consciousness as a natural sensibility. This mutability amidst presumed naturalness makes race a central tactic of crisis production and containment for the capitalist state. Melamed does justice to a critical feature of racial capitalist statecraft that is missing from most insta-simplistic critiques of racial capitalism: whiteness is fungible. In the so-called Progressive Era, the wages of whiteness shifted shape in what Melamed calls "the multicultural phase of neoliberal racial capitalism."[38]

---

37. Julia Buxton, *The Political Economy of Narcotics: Production, Consumption and Global Markets* (London: Zed Books, 2006).
38. Jodi Melamed, *Represent and Destroy: Rationalizing Violence in the New Racial Capitalism* (Minneapolis: University of Minnesota Press, 2011).

Shifting regimes of capital formation accompany shifting regimes of meaning-making. For example, we can see how neoliberalism changed the contours of the logics and regimes of "official" racial order. Melamed says, "Privileged and stigmatized racial formations no longer mesh perfectly with a color line. Instead, new categories of privilege and stigma determined by ideological, economic, and cultural criteria overlay older, conventional racial categories, so that traditionally recognized racial identities—Black, Asian, white, or Arab/Muslim—can now occupy both sides of the privilege/stigma opposition."[39]

We can see and reckon with capital's capacity to renovate existing social formations of inequality, race central among them, for its changing purposes. In the neoliberal era, all blue-collar workers were denigrated, and new stories were needed to maintain the state of things. The (formally/formerly) white, blue-collar working class, once essential to American capitalism's unified self-concept, were disciplined with debt and reproduced in the national-liberal story as deplorable criminal-addicts, derelict and lazy, deserving of being discarded. These stories are of a piece with shame-based morality tales long used by 'free market' reformers to characterize poor, Black Americans. "I have known many welfare queens," writes JD Vance in his *Hillbilly Elegy*, "some were my neighbors, and all were white."[40]

GOD, THE DEVIL, AND SHAME

The policing of unruly bodies, the produced and ongoing fracturing of our sense of self as separate and divided, internally and externally, is an incoherent and necessary instrument of domination and accumulation, and a central causal feature of disordered consumption-based coping mechanisms. Shame is a central apparatus, a technology of imperial rule, that allows for the inner dimensions of colonized, partitioned consciousness. Shame and its discounting of self and self-worth, are central to the collective construct of the "addict."

---

39. Jodi Melamed, "The Spirit of Neoliberalism: From Racial Liberalism to Neoliberal Multiculturalism," *Social Text* 24, no. 4 (2006): 1–24.
40. J.D. Vance, *Hillbilly Elegy: A Memoir of a Family and Culture in Crisis* (New York: Harper, 2016).

In the opioid crisis, even in the "kinder, gentler" medical model, shame is central to the containment strategy of carceral interventions, even "compassionate-carceral" (like compulsory rehab for the indigent and treatment facilities within prisons) fixes to the problem of mass dependency. The carceral state seeks not to resolve the crisis of deleterious use and dependence but to contain, by punishment and removal, those whose use spills over into the public sphere.

Drug use and shame are often concurrent conditions. Drug use is often pushed on populations who are dominated, and shame about use can then be deployed to blame conquered people for their suffering. In *Flesh and Stone* (1996), Richard Sennett states the matter plainly: "Any society needs strong moral sanctions to make people tolerate, much less experience positively, duality, incompleteness, and otherness. Moral sanctions arose in Western civilization through the powers of religion."[41] This strategy has the added benefit of being "postracial."[42]

Shame is a technology of partition in the human consciousness that supersedes racial logics of partition but is *put to work* by racial and racist regimes of capital's empire. Shame undergirds the present paradigm's partitions of "deserving" and "undeserving." The shape-shifting construct known as the "addict" reveals how shame, always entangled with racialized logics of failure and inhumanity, remains a central tactic of capitalist ideological governance. Shame is baked into liberal social control, with the state's doubling down on liberalism's and bourgeoise economics' founding myth of self-reliance, animated by the specter of *Homo economicus*. Shame is central to the carceral containment strategy of neoliberalism's inherent social fallout; it is a redoubled and clandestine tactic to render culpable (and inferior) those whose suffering, were it to be recognized as structural, preventable, and for another (class)'s gain, would incriminate the social order and threaten a legitimacy crisis.

Shame factors like an invisible weapon in all manner of institutions in the service of maintaining the status quo. Like Marx says of value, shame is immaterial but objective. We know when shame is present, even if it remains unseen to the eye. In the previously

---

41. Richard Sennett, *Flesh and Stone*, 374.
42. Melamed, *The Spirit of Neoliberalism* (2006) and *Represent and Destroy* (2011).

redacted court documents made available in the 2019 Commonwealth of Massachusetts versus Purdue and Sackler case, Richard Sackler, Arthur's nephew, who became president of Purdue in 1999 and served as Chairman of the Board until 2007, is quoted as saying the litigation strategy should focus on the lack of credibility of the "addicted" plaintiff, instructing the legal team to "hammer on the abusers in every way possible."[43] This strategy proved very successful in courtrooms across the country. Purdue's defense won individual and class-level cases by discrediting the plaintiff as derelict, shifty, and drug-seeking, painting them as uncredible witness to the events of their own life.

To perpetuate relational ways of being that condemn people who do not *behave rationally* is to tell a limiting and conscripting lie about what it is to be a human being at all.[44] It illustrates precisely that rationality and reason are disciplinary apparatuses, confining our consciousness, appealing to our lower cognitive functioning, our fear of being cast out and condemned. We are social animals, a part of the entangled web of rebellious life. Embracing this fact is central to our collective salvation. Shame is central to "obedience" in imperialist social formations because being cast out from the group is still a fate as bad as, or assuring of, death in our biological survival imprinting.

Shame is such an effective strategy for dislocating the crisis because it is both a predictor of drug use and a weapon to disavow, punish, abandon, and blame those who use drugs. Shame's logic is circular and slippery. It is a powerful weapon in imperialism's toolbox because of how easily it grafts onto our lower-order evolutionary brain circuitry. Being primates and interdependent creatures, belonging is essential to our survival. The paradigm deploys shame as a strategy of partition. When we are defending our very worthiness or right to exist—or worse, when we believe the paradigm's lie of our unworthiness—we are conscripted to play the system's domination games.

---

43. *Commonwealth of Massachusetts v. Purdue Pharma L.P., Purdue Pharma Inc., Richard Sackler, Theresa Sackler, et. al.*, January 31, 2019, https://www.mass.gov/files/documents/2019/07/11/43_01%20First%20Amended%20Complaint%20filed%2001-31-2019_0.pdf; Barry Meier, "Origins of an Epidemic: Purdue Pharma Knew Its Opioids Were Widely Abused," *New York Times*, May 29, 2018, sec. Health, https://www.nytimes.com/2018/05/29/health/purdue-opioids-OxyContin.html.
44. Douglas Crimp, *Melancholia and Moralism: Essays on AIDS and Queer Politics* (Cambridge, MA: MIT Press, 2004).

As former Black Panther and incarcerated person Michael "Cetewayo" Tabor put it in *Capitalism Plus Dope Equals Genocide* (1969), "These feelings of inferiority gave birth to a sense of self-hatred which finds expression in self-destructive behavior patterns. The wretchedness of our plight, our sense of powerlessness and despair created within our minds a predisposition toward the use of any substance which produced euphoric illusions."[45]

Shame is a central affective tactic that undergirds mass incarceration and the dehumanization and cognitive dissonance required for the human labor that animates every circuit of the present-day system where social problems are answered with cops, courts, and cages. It is the internalized articulation of external oppression, the belief not that one has done badly but that one is bad, and is co-constitutive with a negative self-concept and perception of self in relation to other(s) and the collective whole.[46]

The lie of *Homo economicus* shapes the contours of our political consciousness, constructing collective notions of whose pain is legitimate, about whose suffering is noble and whose is unseemly, and about who is deserving of help and who must be punished. Chris Hedges and Joe Sacco observe shame as a tactic of warfare, imperial repression, and crowd control in their reflections on the Pine Ridge reservation in *Days of Destruction, Days of Revolt*.[47] Self-loathing and self-harm, imposed through structurally inflicted trauma and regimental dehumanization, produce populations who police themselves, whose very self-concept has been colonized. It is an insurance policy against revolt.

---

45. Michael "Cetewayo" Tabor, *Capitalism Plus Dope Equals Genocide*, nd, https://www.marxists.org/history/usa/workers/black-panthers/1970/dope.htm.
46. Krista Tippett, "Bessel van der Kolk—How Trauma Lodges in the Body," *On Being with Krista Tippett*, December 19, 2019, https://www.npr.org/sections/money/2010/08/03/128960709/the-tuesday-podcast; Bessel van der Kolk, *The Body Keeps the Score: Brain, Mind, and Body in the Healing of Trauma* (New York: Penguin Books, 2015).
47. Chris Hedges and Joe Sacco, *Days of Destruction, Days of Revolt* (New York: Bold Type Books, 2014).

THE DISLOCATION THEORY OF ADDICTION

Numbers vary depending on study and substance, but the data on drug use versus dependence handedly refutes the commodity-fetish based story of the irresistible allure of dependency-forming substances, sometimes called the 'demon drug' myth. My friend Peter, a homeless man who injects opioids, told me his story. He was a unionized carpenter and made a good living, had good benefits and was building a solid pension. He had a wife and family, two teenage daughters. In the late 1990s, his twin teenage daughters begged him for braces to "correct" their crooked teeth. I was not above this kind of socialization of desire or the compulsion to conform to market-sized standards of beauty and femininity. I too mistook crooked teeth correction as a need, and I smile my straightened-toothed smile at Peter when he shares this, confessing that I too lobbied my parents for braces in the late 1990s, to "correct" what my brother Joe always teased was a *snaggle tooth*.

Peter picked up some weekend work under the table to pay the insurance copayment for the orthodontist. You can tell by the way he says it that the amount felt extortionist. Through a thick Maine accent and Irish ancestral gift for delightfully performative storytelling, he exclaims, "*Fooah-thousand dollahs!*" The way he says it also lets me know that he had a habit of indulging his daughters, and I say so, which makes us both laugh. "Oh, wrapped around their little fingers, totally," he says as we giggle together.

One Saturday morning, on a side job earning money for his daughters' braces, Peter fell through the floor on the second story of a building and straight to the concrete on the ground floor. The fall shattered several vertebrae in his lower back and broke his femur. He was given opioids for the pain. He was out of work for a long time, but since the injury was sustained outside his unionized job, he was disqualified for workers compensation insurance. Bills piled up. Pills filled the void. The rest, his present state tells it, is history. When he was prescribed opioids, no one asked, and he didn't offer, that he was an old acquaintance of the morphine molecule. At eighteen years old, he found himself in a difficult situation and the substance offered some relief. Drafted to fight in Vietnam, Peter, along with an estimated 40 percent of deployed soldiers, regularly used heroin to take the edge off a reality too painful to bear.[48]

Heroin has long been considered an antidote against fear—or at least, for all sensations relating to fear and its relatives: pain, grief, and despair. A report in *The New York Times* from May 16, 1971 begins: "The use of heroin by American troops in Vietnam has reached epidemic proportions."[49] Defense Department studies indicated that 43 percent of returning soldiers admitted to using narcotics while deployed and half of those reported becoming dependent.[50] The heroin market in Southeast Asian countries swelled as a result of the war, in part due to explicit pacts with heroin-producing cadres in the region by the CIA.[51] The Drug Enforcement Administration was established on July 1, 1973. Among its founding mandates was the problem of growing heroin use among American soldiers deployed in Vietnam.

In his book *The Globalization of Addiction*, psychologist Bruce Alexander posits that addiction is an adaptation to "psychosocial dislocation."[52] Borrowing economic historian Karl Polanyi's term, "dislocation" refers to the upheaval inherent in the imposition and penetration of capitalist market relations and the fact that the profit motive destroys existing social and environmental relations. Alexander draws a connection between constant ongoing upheaval, not only as market logics penetrate new places but new sectors of our lives, and the rising instance of disordered drug consumption. In the production of human beings as rational economic actors, purpose, meaning, social ties, and connection to place are categorically torn asunder. Addictions, Alexander says, are a substitute for psychosocial

---

48.　Lee N. Robins et al., "Vietnam Veterans Three Years after Vietnam: How Our Study Changed Our View of Heroin," *American Journal on Addictions* 19, no. 3 (May 1, 2010): 203–211; Alfred W. McCoy, *The Politics of Heroin in Southeast Asia* (New York: Harper & Row, 1972).

49.　Alvin M. Shuster, "G.I. Heroin Addiction Epidemic in Vietnam," *New York Times*, May 16, 1971, sec. Archives, https://www.nytimes.com/1971/05/16/archives/gi-heroin-addiction-epidemic-in-vietnam-gi-heroin-addiction-is.html.

50.　Lee N. Robins, Darlene H. Davis, and David N. Nurco, "How Permanent Was Vietnam Drug Addiction?," *American Journal of Public Health* 64, no. 12 (December 1974): 38–43; Robins et al., "Vietnam Veterans Three Years after Vietnam."

51.　Alfred McCoy, *The Politics of Heroin: CIA Complicity in the Global Drug Trade* (Chicago: Lawrence Hill Books, 2003); Alfred McCoy, *The Politics of Heroin in Southeast Asia* (New York: Harper and Row, 1972); Booth, *Opium: A History*.

52.　Bruce K. Alexander, *The Globalization of Addiction: A Study in Poverty of the Spirit* (New York: Oxford University Press, 2008).

integration. In other words, drug use in commodity-centric cultures substitutes for connection.

A longitudinal US Department of Defense study on returning Vietnam soldiers found that 20 percent of returning enlisted men by 1975 met the diagnostic criteria for heroin addiction. Critically—remission rates one year after returning home were found to be 95 percent, "unheard of among narcotic addicts treated in the U.S."[53] This proved to be a powerful finding, given the demon-commodity narrative so commonly spun about drugs in general and heroin in particular— that people become hooked after one use. The case of heroin use and dependence among US soldiers in Vietnam echoes Alexander's dislocation theory of addiction—that drug use is a coping mechanism for the loss or lack of psychosocial integration.[54]

Rather than a brain disease, moral scourge, or the totalizing allure of the substance itself, the experience of American soldiers' consumption patterns in and upon returning home from Vietnam demonstrates that consumption of commodified relief is an adaptive strategy for survival amidst unlivable circumstances. The researchers on the Vietnam study learned that of those 5 percent of dependent veterans who continued using at home some commonalities presented themselves. In general, the men were found to have been significantly more likely to have come home to insufficient networks of support—job and family, as well as being more likely to have experienced traumatic events earlier in life, before active combat.[55]

Health, like wealth, is unequally distributed in the present world dis-order. At the individual and the societal level, the significant relationship between stress and addiction has been definitively demonstrated. Studies also demonstrate substance use disorder to be more

53.   Robins, Davis, and Nurco, "How Permanent Was Vietnam Drug Addiction?"; Lee N. Robins, "Vietnam Veterans' Rapid Recovery from Heroin Addiction: A Fluke or Normal Expectation?," *Addiction* 88, no. 8 (August 1993): 1041–1054.
54.   Bruce Alexander is often called a Canadian psychologist, but I learned in personal conversation with him—when I arranged for him to deliver the keynote address at the 2015 Maine Harm Reduction Alliance Annual Conference and had the pleasure of driving him from Portland to Lewiston for the event—that he's an American who fled to Canada as a young man in order to evade being drafted to fight in the Vietnam War.
55.   Sally Satel and Scott O. Lilienfeld, "Addiction and the Brain Disease Fallacy," from *Brainwashed: The Seductive Appeal of Mindless Neuroscience* (New York: Basic Books, 2013)

prevalent in societies with higher rates of economic inequality.[56] "Addicts" perform an enormously important role for the maintenance of the system, allowing capitalism's embedded harms to be offshored and outsourced into the cognitive-embodied spirits of the ever-growing numbers of human beings on the losing end of the equation.

Gabor Maté says, "Addictions always originate in pain. The question is not 'why the addiction?' but 'why the pain?'"[57] The data bears conclusive evidence that childhood trauma, traumatic experience in early life, or, being gestated in the womb of a mother who lives with a preponderance of fear, is a significant determinant to health and well-being outcomes, including propensity for drug dependence and behavioral addictions.[58] Childhood exposure to extreme chronic stress and traumatic experiences produces adult dysfunction in the form of emotional dysregulation and limited capacity for self-soothing, aggression against self and others, dissociation from one's physical body or sense of self, attention problems, a host of physical health issues, and difficulties with self-concept and in maintaining satisfactory interpersonal relationships.

The results of the first Adverse Childhood Experiences (ACE) study, released in 1998, examined over 18,000 health records and found that childhood trauma and household dysfunction were significant precursors to a range of health problems, including addiction and premature death in adulthood.[59] Rather than personal pathology, bad genes, or bad choices the ACE study demonstrates that inequality, poverty, maternal stress, and violent environments (including the prevalence of policing and carceral-state intervention) matters in the development of the brain, nervous system, and embodied psyche of young children and that the impacts persist into adulthood. Adverse

56. Richard Wilkinson and Kate Pickett, *The Spirit Level: Why Greater Equality Makes Societies Stronger* (New York: Bloomsbury Publishing, 2011); Richard Wilkinson and Kate Pickett, *The Inner Level: How More Equal Societies Reduce Stress, Restore Sanity and Improve Everyone's Well-Being* (New York: Penguin Press, 2019).

57. Gabor Maté, *Scattered Minds: The Origins and Healing of Attention Deficit Disorder* (Toronto: Vermilion, 2019).

58. Laurence Heller and Aline LaPierre, *Healing Developmental Trauma: How Early Trauma Affects Self-Regulation, Self-Image, and the Capacity for Relationship* (Berkeley: North Atlantic Books, 2012); Steven N. Gold, *Not Trauma Alone: Therapy for Child Abuse Survivors in Family and Social Context* (Philadelphia: Routledge, 2000).

59. V. J. Felitti et al., "Relationship of Childhood Abuse and Household Dysfunction to Many of the Leading Causes of Death in Adults. The Adverse Childhood Experiences (ACE) Study," *American Journal of Preventive Medicine* 14, no. 4 (May 1998): 245–258.

childhood experiences shape not only perceptions of self, other, and greater contexts, but the physical contours of the brain, and other spatial, embodied, synaptic circuitry of the human organism, most notably the nervous system.

ACEs are additive and they exponentially increase the risks of substance use disorder, as well as other kinds of physical and mental illness. Studies using the ACE framework have corroborated that a high prevalence of ACEs strongly predicts the disordered use of psychoactive substances in adulthood.[60] For each adverse childhood experience, data suggest a two-to-fourfold increased risk of the adoption of substance-based coping mechanisms in early adulthood. Subjects with five or more ACEs had seven to ten times greater risk than did those with none.[61]

Other frameworks beyond the ACE study also demonstrate that stressful environments during one's upbringing correlates significantly to health outcomes in adulthood. For example, in her book *Scared Sick* (2012), Robin Karr-Morse integrates research from psychology, neurobiology, endocrinology, immunology, and genetics to demonstrate that chronic fear in infancy and early childhood predispose adult illnesses, including substance use disorder.[62] Nervous system dysregulation and general malaise and dis-ease are on a continuum with traumatic stress, unmourned grief, and other kinds of stuck, unprocessed pain, all of which lead people to seek relief where and how they can, within the means and the limits of their budgets, environments, and imaginaries (the canvas for producing possible strategies) that are available to us.

---

60. Robert F. Anda et al., "Adverse Childhood Experiences, Alcoholic Parents, and Later Risk of Alcoholism and Depression," *Psychiatric Services* 53, no. 8 (August 2002): 1001–1009; Shanta R. Dube et al., "Exposure to Abuse, Neglect, and Household Dysfunction among Adults Who Witnessed Intimate Partner Violence as Children: Implications for Health and Social Services," *Violence and Victims* 17, no. 1 (February 2002): 3–17.

61. Gabor Maté, *In the Realm of Hungry Ghosts: Close Encounters with Addiction* (Berkeley: North Atlantic Books, 2011).

62. Robin Karr-Morse and Meredith S. Wiley, *Scared Sick: The Role of Childhood Trauma in Adult Disease* (New York: Basic Books, 2012).

COMMODITY FETISHISM AND SO-CALLED "DEMON DRUGS"

A commodity is produced in some quantity for sale on a market. It is valuable precisely for its lack of specificity, that it appears "out of nowhere," as if without history or context, and with no consideration for the human hands or Earth-based inputs that summoned it into existence.

Commodity fetishism names the fact that market-based social provision in the form of commodity production makes us all forget that making, producing, sharing, and consuming things is a social relation and a relational unity. More than anything, it is this inherent relationality, interdependence, place-based communal fact of consumption, production, distribution, and exchange that capitalist consciousness and its partitioning myth of separate, individual, and unequal must evade in order to exist.

The "demon drugs" perspective on addiction attributes almost supernatural powers to substances, compelling individuals into addiction, which can be seen as a manifestation of commodity fetishism. The focus on the all-powerful substances themselves obscures the underlying social, economic, and psychological factors that contribute to addiction.

Commodity fetishism involves ascribing inherent value or power to objects, independent of the social relations that give rise to them. Similarly, the demon drug theory elevates substances to a position of autonomous power, disregarding the complex interplay of societal structures, individual vulnerabilities, and broader economic forces. By doing so, it not only mystifies the nature of addiction but also inadvertently contributes to the stigmatization of individuals struggling with substance use, reducing their experience to a simplistic interaction with a "demonic" commodity, rather than a multifaceted health issue embedded in a broader socioeconomic context.

THE VALUE OF THE "ADDICT"

What does the "addict" hide? What does the construct explain away that needs interrogation? Toni Morrison's 1995 speech, "Racism and Fascism" contains a ten-point plan for fascist control, the first of which is, "Construct an internal enemy, as both focus and diversion."[63] The story of the so-called "addict" illustrates the state strategy to make an internal enemy both a focus and a diversion. In American political history, the "addict" has been renovated in scope, understanding, and tenor, a process which belies a recognizable pattern wherein a denigrated category of human being is produced or deployed in order to contain critique that would destabilize the ruling authority's legitimacy. In this case, the "addict" *fixes* the problem of mass suffering, geographically locates the narrative at the level of the individuals in question. If the people suffering can be said to be themselves the reason for their suffering, critique and questioning of the system is curtailed. The "addict" performs an embodied spatial fix, bears a burden of causality for the system's inherent unevenness in social suffering.

Marxist feminist scholars render visible the *value* of denigrated and reduced categories of humanity to the capitalist system, given its existential need for partition and social hierarchy.[64]

For example, Melissa Wright focuses her analysis on maquiladora workers in Mexico but we see it everywhere we see large-scale industrial production historically and today, from the Triangle factory fire in New York City in the early twentieth century, to the garment factory collapses in Bangladesh in 2011, to the labor conditions we learn about at Foxconn factories—where women laborers are fired for becoming pregnant and are forced to sign paperwork promising that they will not commit suicide, because it's bad for publicity and therefore stock prices.[65]

Wright's intervention is more nuanced and useful than simply "capitalism destroys women." She reminds us that in their production as *lesser than human*, women industrial workers are invaluable to capitalism, precisely because their degradation allows for extremely high rates of surplus value extraction to be stolen from them. The

63. Toni Morrison, "Racism and Fascism" (lecture delivered at Howard University, March 3, 1995), *The Journal of Negro Education* 64, no. 3 (1995): 384–390.

64. Maria Mies, *Patriarchy and Accumulation on a World Scale: Women in the International Division of Labour* (London: Zed Books, 1999); J. K. Gibson-Graham, *A Postcapitalist Politics* (Minneapolis: University of Minnesota Press, 2006).

65. Chris Fraser, "iPhone Factory Revolt: What's Next After Police Beatings of Chinese Workers Protesting Wages, COVID Policy," *Toronto Star*, November 24, 2022, https://www. thestar.com/news/world/iphone-factory-revolt-whats-next-after-police-beatings-of-chinese-workers-protesting-wages-covid-policy/article_da2878b1-5883-51ad-91ba-7b31c1e750a4.html.

condition of rising rates of exploitation, central to today's global capitalism, requires not merely the disposal or extermination of marked groups of humans, but their entrenchment in a slow death, a position of no future, no alternative, no dignity, no humanity.[66] Capital's quest for endless growth necessitates a state apparatus capable of producing increasing populations and places from which the system's agents can produce extraction in perpetuity.

Competing formations for state control use the fact of drugs and dependence in their existential quest to produce an internal and external threat, that which allows the state's monopoly on violence. Ideological formations of group-differentiated lesser subjectivities, through racial and other categories, "the addict" among them, attempt to produce cognitive dissonance and passive consent to the ongoingness of social harm. They aim to train a general populace not to recognize structural and preventable harm, or to sell a saleable narrative that a witnessed harm is self-inflicted or deserved. By cognitively partitioning a collective we into an *us versus them*, control regimes convince us that mass suffering is not a generalizable concern or evidence of systemic injustice.

THE WISDOM IN GETTING HIGH

As capitalist consciousness produces a continual departure from the real, it leaves humans to suffer its embedded harms in its wake. Stuck in place, we inhabit a three-dimensional reality that contradicts our (acknowledged or unacknowledged) desire for life to be lived otherwise. Drug use is a temporary transit from a present reality that reminds the user of other possible realities, as simple as a feeling state, a shift in mind/body perception away. Drug use to escape pain connects one with their essence, the signal behind all the noise of fear, pain and other difficult, trapped feelings. As a flight from space-time, it is a survival strategy, a rebellion against a given, embodied here-and-now

---

66. This echoes Achille Mbembe's intervention in *Necropolitics*. Speaking to Foucault's idea of biopolitics, Mbembe reminds us that the maintenance of the dead but dominant word disorder is more nuanced than the partition of who can live and who must die, but also about who must live in degraded circumstances, a condition in which some even can then produce a capitalist-as-savior narrative for giving them work at all. The argument is also resonant with Giorgio Agamben's argument in *Homo Sacer: Sovereign Power and Bare Life*.

that has been produced as painful and unmanageable. The European imperial project which birthed contemporary capitalism was simultaneously a project to conquer and discipline human concepts of both space and time. Among the many ways human consciousness was dominated by imperial conquest was the instantiation of abstracted, mathematical clock time as the only system by which time was made to be meaningful.[67] Ann Marlowe's 2000 memoir of heroin addiction is seductively titled *How to Stop Time*.[68] Martin Booth, in the introduction to his book *Opium* (1998) says, "To an addict, opium and its derivatives are the raw substance of dreams, the means of escape from reality and temporary entry into heaven—or at least *another place apart from the here and now*."[69]

Clementine Morrigan argues for a conceptualization of addiction, and other self-harming behaviors, summed up in what they call "acting out" as "an embodied form of testimony."[70] Morrigan, a self-identifying "sober alcoholic,'" defines alcoholism as "an inverted quest for magic." Silvia Federici's rejoinder to *Caliban and the Witch, Re-enchanting the World* from 2019 reminds us that recovering from the lifeless paradigm entails a quest to feel the magic of aliveness that capital's linear logics and pursuit of profit stomp out.[71] Addiction provides the rituals, customs, sense of purpose, and definition to a life otherwise absent of other meaningful (nonpainful) social connections. Physiological dependence can be a component of an addiction, and certainly is one in the case of opioids and opiates, but the phenomenon of addiction, or substance use disorder, is not reducible to physiological dependence. Addiction is the habituation of a substance or behavior pursued in hopes of achieving "flight from distress."[72] Behavioral patterning and the ritualized nature of dependent consumption is central. Dr. Daniel Sumrok, director of the Center for Addiction Sciences at the University of Tennessee Health Science Center's College of

---

67. Giordano Nanni, *The Colonisation of Time: Ritual, Routine and Resistance in the British Empire* (Manchester: Manchester University Press, 2012).
68. Ann Marlowe, *How to Stop Time: Heroin from A To Z* (New York: Basic Books, 1999).
69. Martin Booth, *Opium: A History* (New York: St. Martin's Press, 1998), xii. Emphasis added.
70. Clementine Morrigan, *Trauma Magic* (Clementine Morrigan, 2017).
71. Silvia Federici, *Re-Enchanting the World: Feminism and the Politics of the Commons* (Oakland: PM Press, 2019).
72. Maté, *In the Realm of Hungry Ghosts*, 17.

Medicine says, "Addiction shouldn't be called 'addiction.' It should be called 'ritualized compulsive comfort-seeking.'"[73]

In a commodity-based economic system driven by the quest to accumulate wealth, the consumption of commodities is presented as the first-order solution to most problems. The annihilation of space by time means also the annihilation of the body and the instantiation of a fear-based relational way of knowing, a severed and isolated sense of self in relation to the whole, amidst consciousness steeped in scarcity and a sense of pervasive looming threat.[74] Capitalism's irrationality, "the madness of economic reason" to use Harvey's phrase, spreads to all social relations, including the relationships between humans and the bodies of water and land that sustain our very life.[75]

Commodity fetishism is utterly central to the production of ways of seeing and understanding drug use and habituation. Fetishizing the supposed siren song of demonic commodity drugs ("one hit and you're *hooked*" narratives, like those sold en masse to American children in Nancy Reagan's Just Say No initiative), allows for the dehumanization of those who fall under their spell and allows for the animation of state and market-based policies of extermination, abandonment, and dehumanized containment. Addiction is not about the commodities in question around which an individual may choose to self-soothe. It is a journey from the present and the spacetime of the body in its given context to a more hopeful, playful, connected, knowing—remembering against the forced forgetting, imagining against the many conscripted cognitive foreclosures.

Drug use can be practice for life, unless and until it becomes a substitute for living. Drug use can help one anchor in the feeling state of *feeling good*. In taking temporary transit to a place where pain subsides and magic resides, we can remember deeper truths that pain and threat drown out. We can connect to purpose and possibility, two things every human needs, and, possibly, learn to build bridges that

---

73. Jane Allen Stevens, "Addiction Doc Says It's Not the Drugs, It's Adverse Childhood Experiences," *Social Justice Solutions*, September 29, 2017, https://www.socialjusticesolutions.org/2017/09/29/addiction-doc-says-not-drugs-adverse-childhood-experiences/.

74. Donald M. Lowe, *The Body in Late-Capitalist USA* (Durham: Duke University Press, 1995); David Harvey, "The Body as an Accumulation Strategy," *Environment and Planning D: Society and Space* 16, no. 4 (August 1998): 401–421.

75. David Harvey, *Marx, Capital, and the Madness of Economic Reason* (New York: Oxford University Press, 2017).

allow us to access such states in our so-called ordinary consciousness. Ritualized comfort-seeking with commodity substances stands in—in a commodity-driven, alienated world—for the rituals and comforts of belonging, of remembering our ancestors' traditions and cosmologies, like honoring the seasons and the stars and the Earth, our living source of life.

Dopamine is released in pursuit of what we deem to have meaning. It is not the attainment but the seeking that releases this (to oversimplify in layperson's terms) "pleasure" chemical. The quest for purpose and meaning is innate to the species. Capital's empire co-opts it, like it does every human impulse. Maté observes a similar spirit in his patients in Vancouver's Downtown Eastside neighborhood and corroborates it with latest fMRI-based neuroscience on addiction:

> The wondrous power of a drug is to offer the addict protection from pain while at the same time enabling her to engage the world with excitement and meaning. 'It's not that my senses are dulled—no, they open, expanded' explained a young woman whose substances of choice are cocaine and marijuana. 'But the anxiety is removed, and the nagging guilt and—yeah!' The drug restores to the addict the childhood vivacity she suppressed long ago.[76]

Despair characterizes addiction and alienation. New histories for new theories, storytelling that changes our sight, can be an antidote to all of these. Connection to our felt senses and perceptual capacities, through drugs or other kinds of altered states of consciousness, can allow us to identify the cracks in the wall that are portals to other dimensions, an expanded reality, way of seeing and knowing and contextualizing the present, the fertile ground from which we can collectively dream of other possible futures.

Drug use, then, is a rational response to an irrational way of life. Disordered use is a reasonable response to a disordered society. Consumption-based transit from the here and now is a likely approach in a consumption-based framework rife with incessant cognitive-embodied squeezes, and sped-up foreclosure of life chances. Cindi Katz reminds us that the "scale of dispossession is witnessed not just in

---

76. Maté, *In the Realm of Hungry Ghosts*, 41.

uneven geographical developments like colonialism, gentrification, suburbanization, or "urban renewal," but also at the intimate scales of everyday life. Foreclosure takes place—quite literally—at the very heart of people's existence."[77] Individuals with a propensity to self-soothe through substance consumption often have limited resources for restoring a sense of emotional or socio-spatial balance. There are several reasons for this, but they all boil down to unhealed emotional wounding (trauma) coupled with a lack of available alternatives for healing or relief.

Columbia University professor and neurobiologist Carl Hart counters the demon-drug narrative with evidence to support crack cocaine use as an economically rational choice.[78] In a series of experiments offering users of crack and methamphetamine who did not wish to quit choices between varying size doses of their drug of choice and money or cash vouchers, Hart and his research team concluded that users make economically rational choices. Typically, the research found that users would choose a $5 reward rather than small doses of crack, but preferred the crack when the dose was larger. When offered $20 to forgo using, regardless of the size of the dose, subjects chose the money every time, refuting commonplace perception perpetuated by Nancy Reagan's Just Say No and other 'awareness' campaigns in the eighties of the user who can't stop once they get a taste. "When they were given an alternative to crack, they made rational economic decisions," Hart said to a journalist with the *Huffington Post* about the findings.[79] Hart points out that the hysteria around drugs and drug users goes unchallenged because it is embedded in the funding streams and missions of the existing institutions and insufficient paradigms for addressing disordered drug use, saying in the same interview, "We spend $26 billion a year on the drug war. Law enforcement and prisons get a large amount of money to continue to perpetuate this stuff

77.   Cindi Katz, "Accumulation, Excess, Childhood: Toward a Countertopography of Risk and Waste," *Documents d'Analisi Geografica* 57, no. 1 (2011): 47–60.

78.   Carl Hart, *High Price: A Neuroscientist's Journey of Self-Discovery That Challenges Everything You Know About Drugs and Society* (New York: HarperCollins, 2013); John Tierney, "The Rational Choices of Crack Addicts," *New York Times*, September 16, 2013, sec. Science, https://www.nytimes.com/2013/09/17/science/the-rational-choices-of-crack-addicts.html.

79.   Simon McCormack, "Drug Addicts Make Rational Choices, Scientist Argues," *Huffington Post*, September 19, 2013, https://www.huffpost.com/entry/drug-addicts-make-rational-choices_n_3955171.

. . ." adding, "researchers, treatment providers—we all have a stake in the drug hysteria game."

Carl Hart's experiment regarding "rational choice" and drug users can be extended to consider the rational choice to subvert, stretch, and depart from linear clock time. In line with this, Nick Reding's *Methland* chronicles working-class methamphetamine use and its widespread adoption in parts of the country where union busting, agglomeration, automation, and a coordinated switch to recruiting undocumented laborers in labor-intensive farming and processing jobs led to the decimation of working-class livelihoods.[80] Meth consumption was for many a rational choice effort to stretch time, to make a day's potential for earning a wage more capacious by staving off the body's need for sleep and rest. Regimes of extraction beget auto-extraction, with a space-time horizon of an ever-faster passing now. We steal from our well-being and extract from our embodiment's future for the sake of earning enough to get by in a rigged system today. Similarly, our relations to other humans, living beings and the Earth mimic the extractivist patterns of capital's aims, as its logics envelop and invert all other aims and intentions. In the words of Ruth Wilson Gilmore, "where life is precious, life is precious,"[81] and where profit is precious, life is cheap. Drug use is a transit to a here-and-now with more connection and less pain for those whose lives and labor have been devalued.

WHAT "ADDICTS" KNOW

Drug use is not about the allure of demon drugs, nor about a desire to die or self-harm. More than anything, an individual's habituated and disordered use of drugs is about a desire or need to traverse the present in a quantum leap while lacking other options for accessing a more livable timeline, spacetime, mindset, and material reality. Drug use as a coping strategy is in some essential way about a hope for an alternative spacetime. The embodied consciousness that people who

---

80. Nick Reding, *Methland: The Death and Life of an American Small Town* (New York: Bloomsbury USA, 2010).
81. Rachel Kushner, "Is Prison Necessary? Ruth Wilson Gilmore Might Change Your Mind," *New York Times*, April 17, 2019, sec. Magazine, https://www.nytimes.com/2019/04/17/magazine/prison-abolition-ruth-wilson-gilmore.html.

self-soothe with drugs access in the state of a drug high is in some essential ways an anchor out of a present consumed with pain and despair into the feeling state of a viable possible future. The feeling state of an opioid high is one of feeling right with life, self, and the world. It is the feeling of being capable, powerful, content, good, and unbothered. Dr. George Wood, in his 1868 volume *A Treatise on Therapeutics and Pharmacology or Materia Medica*, describes it by saying, "It seems to make the individual, for the time, a better and greater man."[82] Drug use in this light is a strategy born of a choice to survive what feels, for good reasons, unlivable.

The case for seeing drug use as rational choice mirrors the intervention made by Marxist political ecologist Piers Blaikie in his 1985 *The Political Ecology of Soil Erosion in Developing Countries*.[83] As a subfield within the critical social sciences, political ecology examines the political and economic dynamics that drive seemingly irrational choices among farmers, foresters, and other stewards of the living Earth. Blaikie's work rejected the existing science of soil erosion that found causal explanation in determinist, Malthusian presumptions of overpopulation and irrational, "backward" actors. Blaikie demonstrated that the depletion of the soil was in fact a rational action. In response to being taxed, exploited and extracted from, peasant farmers in turn extracted from and taxed the land through "irrational" heavy and short-sighted pesticide and fertilizer use. Blaikie framed his research in terms of *maladaptation*, drawing on cases where land conservation efforts were failing. Focusing on the relations of production for peasant producers, Blaikie demonstrated that continued soil erosion could be explained as a rational behavioral response from peasants: "peasants destroy their own environments in attempts to delay their own destruction."[84]

Carl Hart's intervention, seen in the light of Blaikie's demonstration on the rationality of personally deleterious choices in context, render visible the rationality of survival-based choices amid constant and pressing external threats to survival. We can thus see the often villainized "dope fiend" or compulsive use as an adaptive mechanism of a human organism in pain. Drug use can be seen as an empowered

---

82. Metzger, *Birth of Heroin*, 5.
83. Piers M. Blaikie, *The Political Economy of Soil Erosion in Developing Countries* (London: Routledge, 1985).
84. Blaikie, *The Political Economy of Soil Erosion*, 29.

decision to turn a momentary tide against despair, to take flight from distress, to find agency, relief, and capacity. Research shows that continued use reconfigures neural pathways and brain chemistry making the habituation to use, and so-called relapse, also rational.

Popular myths and political rhetoric often suggest continued drug use is indicative of a desire to die, a suicide in slow motion. A *political ecology* approach, and other perspectives that consider dialectical relationality between individuals and their social environment, allow us to see drug use as indicative of a desire to live otherwise—to stay in the game of life at least for today. The profit motive, as taught in Microeconomics 101, states firms will stay in business so long as they're covering their expenses, even without making a profit, in the hopes that as long as they're maintaining and not incurring losses, they might someday turn a profit. Firms decide to leave the market, to close up shop, if they incur consecutive losses. This is rational choice. In Khalik Allah's 2015 film *Field Niggas*, a documentary film offering intimate portraits of Harlem drug users and street life, a self-declared alcoholic states: "You maintain, or you throw in the towel."[85]

SHORT-TERM/HIGH YIELD AND AUTO-EXTRACTION

Capital's extractivist logics beget auto-extraction and short-term decision-making. We exploit ourselves, treat ourselves the way capitalism taught us to treat the Earth, life, each other. Short-term, profit-seeking orientation permeates every thread of sociality and frames our relationship to nature as well as our own embodied lives. Lakota scholar Nick Estes speaks of the settler colonial ethos of capitalism, the production of a compulsion to "Drive It Like You Stole It."[86] Estes is describing the extractivist mentality of short-term gain despite long-run consequences. In economistic thinking there is no long-run consideration, and the annihilation of space by time means that the ever-encroaching now only factors into considerations regarding extraction and auto-extraction. Like Keynes famously said, "in the long run, we're all dead."

---

85. *Field Niggas*, directed by Khalik Allah (2015; New York: Allah Production), Internet Archive.
86. Nick Estes, *Our History Is the Future: Standing Rock Versus the Dakota Access Pipeline, and the Long Tradition of Indigenous Resistance* (London and New York: Verso, 2019).

In 2014 I gave a talk called "Toward a Historical Materialist The-ory of Addiction," at the annual Historical Materialism conference in London. After my talk, a group of young people approached me to say they enjoyed my remarks and wanted my feedback on a tract they were preparing. The group, based in Birmingham, UK, was inspired to their theory of drug use as an intensification of leisure time by George Caffentzis' work on the refusal to work.[87] In an email exchange, one Birmingham collective member wrote to me, "Our per-spective embraces an Adornoian negativity as the basis for our critique of social forms, enabling us to develop a rather unpalatable approach to drug use which hopes to raise questions about contemporary modes of work refusal and how these intersect with methods of self-destruc-tion." I never saw the finished piece of writing, but I think of their intervention often in relation to Blaikie's notion about pesticide use and the way capital's ever-intensified extraction begets auto-extraction. The intensification of space-time compression begets choices favoring short-term, high-yield modes of embodied, cognitive states of being.

"DIRTY" BRAINS

My handwritten notes from the September 2015 meeting of the City of Portland, Maine Mayor's Overdose Prevention Taskforce give away the tension coursing through my body: "*NOTHING ado about so so much.*" I sit on the mayor's taskforce, among a proliferation of other task-forces meant to signal that the state is responding to the urgency of the crisis when in fact it is not. In addition to the rash of overdoses cor-responding with covert fentanyl coming to town, one of only two detox facilities in the region, affiliated with Mercy Hospital, has just shut-tered their doors citing fiscal insolvency due to low insurance com-pany reimbursement rates. Amid overwhelming unmet need, and in a state of emergency, this is just another meeting on a bureaucrat's daily schedule. Neoliberal governance is mostly a public relations game.

"Well, that's what we mean when we say *clean*; they *do* need to be cleaned. *Addicts have dirty brains, and they need to be scrubbed clean,*"

---

87. George Caffentzis, *In Letters of Blood and Fire: Work, Machines, and the Crisis of Capitalism* (Oakland: PM Press, 2013).

says the speaker with dramatic conviction. He is owner and director of a new for-profit rehab center and the invited guest for today's
installment of the hour-long, monthly meeting. The facilitator, a
Public Health Department manager, by his own admission, has no
experience, familiarity, or passion for the topic. He is pleased to have
found the guest himself, for the first time not outsourcing the agenda
to the mayor's appointees. He declares we will end fifteen minutes
early so that he can make his son's little league game and turns the
meeting over. The recovery entrepreneur describes a program based
in the "confrontational approach" and showcases his own fire-and-
brimstone philosophy of so-called addiction—*the problem is a shameful
lack of self-control; the cure is to be good and not bad.* This is one of the
slews of costly and not at all evidence-based rehab modalities proliferating in the US, and it's described as being "built around punishment
and 'tough love.'"[88] He cites no research, suggests no knowledge of
trauma-informed recovery standards or other emerging best practices
in the field of recovery. He says that the program only admits people
with private health insurance, not Medicaid coverage, and that they
"absolutely do not admit" persons with violent offenses. "We just can't
have violent criminals in the place, end of story."

I am sitting across from fellow harm reduction advocate, opioid
crisis activist, and person in long-term recovery, David Zysk, and we
are aghast. I am legendarily bad at not showing my emotion in a setting like this, but David is doing an even worse job than I am. His face
is red, his mouth puckered. I can see the veins in his neck, and he
is fidgeting with suppressed rage, flicking his pen, shaking his legs,
and wheeling and rocking in his office chair. David and I catch eyes
a dozen times with that spark, as if asking each other—"*Should we
set it off?*"—but alas we don't. We just sit through it. At the end we
go our separate ways, exhausted and distraught. This is that last time
I'll see David. On November 4, 2015 I wake up to a text from a friend,
"Dude OMG David Zysk" accompanied by the broken heart emoji. I
learn at the clinic later that day that David has been found dead in a

---

88. German Lopez, "She Spent More than $110,000 on Drug Rehab. Her Son Still Died,"
Vox, September 3, 2019, https://www.vox.com/policy-and-politics/2019/9/3/20750587/
rehab-drug-addiction-treatment-sean-blake-opioid-epidemic.

South Portland motel room, on his lunch break from the Preble Street Homeless Services Center, from an apparent fentanyl overdose.

"They Talk; We Die," was a slogan of the national opioid epidemic advocacy group, Young People in Recovery (YPR), of which David Zysk was a founding member of the Maine chapter. He was also a fourth-year social work student at the University of Southern Maine, a father to a three-year-old boy, a beloved caseworker and mentor in the homeless veterans' program at Preble Street, and an active member of the Maine Harm Reduction Alliance. He was a passionate, powerful, and heart-centered speaker whom I'd seen captivate audiences in wooden church pews and plastic lecture hall seats across the state. He was the YPR delegate sent to attend a Washington, DC advocacy meeting on the opioid crisis. Other YPR members in attendance told me, David took Obama's drug czar Michael Botticelli to task on the sickening state of federal government inaction on the crisis, saying at the end of the session on the way out the door, "The meetings are nice, man, but we need *money*. We need *action*, which means *money*. We're *dying* up there, man."

THE EURASIAN MAGPIE

I've brought you a mirror. Look at yourself and remember me.

—Rumi, "A Gift to Bring You"

In November 2015, shook by David Zysk's overdose death, I found a very cheap roundtrip plane ticket and decided to take a spur of the moment trip to visit old friends in Sweden. The decision was a deliberate strategy to surround myself in a different lived reality: to jump scale from a present landscape that my overly taxed soul read as a dangerous and painful dead end, and to inject my consciousness with a possible-future imaginary and be reminded of life's, and my own, goodness.

In Maine I got into the habit of paying attention to birds and found myself particularly drawn to members of the corvine species: ravens and crows. In the tops of the tall pines across from my hilltop, attic-floor bedroom window, against a backdrop of a salty shoreline and grey-blue North-Atlantic vista, I watched ravens build a nest and rear and protect their young. In Sweden, a new corvine presented herself to me, a black and white bird with a long, blue-black tail that flashed yellow, green, and purple in the sun. I'd learn this later, since the sun is scarce in Sweden in late November. This is the Eurasian magpie, *Skata* in Swedish, or *Pica pica* in Latin. The first time I noticed the magpie there were five or six or so gathered in a circle on the roadside pavement, surrounding a dead magpie. As I watched them briefly from a slowly passing car window, I noticed an apparent order, some ceremony, to their gathering around the dead bird. I remarked to myself that in my macabre frame of mind, I immediately wanted to call this gathering a funeral, and laughed off my projecting of an emotional state of mourning, anthropomorphizing human ceremonial order, upon the birds. But later I learned that my projection was partly truth.

To watch them in nature, they appear to be somewhat solitary birds going about their own business, but magpies display a complex rage of socially attuned emotions, including grief. They do in fact gather together to acknowledge their dead. When encircled around the deceased member of the collective, they take turns cawing and laying what appear to be wreaths of grass, according to evolutionary biologist and professor at the University of Colorado, Marc Bekoff.[89]

This sociability seems to result from the animal's capacity to perceive themselves as not only a part of a collective, but as distinct, individual members of a collective. "The only species to have passed this test of mirror self-recognition are the Great Apes, dolphins, Eurasian magpie, and elephants. This demonstrates that an animal is able to see itself as distinct in a collective of others (self-aware), one of the main traits underlying empathy and complex sociability."[90]

Empathy is the capacity to see self in an other; to acknowledge an individual or a group of people's suffering. It is not an admission of culpability or responsibility, which people who guard themselves against empathy believe it to be. Empathy, the capacity to honor another's suffering, is the precursor to solidarity, and the antidote to the

---

89. Marc Bekoff, "Animal Emotions, Wild Justice and Why They Matter: Grieving Magpies, a Pissy Baboon, and Empathic Elephants," *Emotion, Space and Society* 2, no. 2 (January 1, 2009): 82–85.
90. Joshua M. Plotnik, Frans B. M. de Waal, and Diana Reiss, "Self-Recognition in an Asian Elephant," *Proceedings of the National Academy of Sciences of the United States of America* 103, no. 45 (November 7, 2006): 17053–17057.

life-threatening epidemic of cognitive dissonance. Empathic intelligence opens us up to the supramaterial sensing space where we feel how injustice, suffering that could be righted, mitigated, made lesser or abolished, tugs at the collective fabric of who and what we are together.

Evolutionary biologists teach us that emotions, feeling states, the capacity for painful feeling states, evolved in animals and humans to improve their chance of survival.[91] In his groundbreaking book on the healing of trauma, *Waking the Tiger*, psychologist Peter Levine offers solutions to resolving the effects of trauma on the human organism by turning toward our instincts, our supra-cognitive animal nature: "It seems that as we distance ourselves farther and farther from our instinctual roots, we have grown to be a species hell-bent on becoming better and better at making life worse and worse. We have been quite 'successful' in distancing ourselves from our vital core."[92] Practically all biomedical-social approaches to the problem of trauma—until Levine and his cohort of somatic-based understandings began emerging in the early 2000s—start from the logical mind and the inherited notion of a separate mind from body, the Cartesian duality that must be undone in the resuscitation of our senses and imaginary for a life beyond the present mess of it.

The abilities to sense, feel, and perceive deeply are evolutionary advancements. The latest research in the mental health field demonstrates that while there is no evidence of genetic predeterminants to so-called addiction or any so-called mental health condition, there *is* evidence that sensitivity is a genetically inherited trait.[93] A propensity for contemplation, deep sensing, perception, creativity, and emotional intelligence, are genetically predisposed. Surviving the dead but dominant world disorder as a person with such traits is a challenge to say the least. Surviving as a sensitive person in the dead and dying world disorder makes one sick.

---

91.   Marc Bekoff, *Animals Matter: A Biologist Explains Why We Should Treat Animals with Compassion and Respect* (Boston: Shambhala Publications, 2007); Marc Bekoff, "Animal Emotions, Wild Justice and Why They Matter: Grieving Magpies, a Pissy Baboon, and Empathic Elephants," *Emotion, Space and Society* 2, no. 2 (January 1, 2009): 82–85.

92.   Peter A. Levine and Ann Frederick, *Waking the Tiger: Healing Trauma* (Berkeley: North Atlantic Books, 1997), 226.

93.   Gabor Maté and Daniel Maté, *The Myth of Normal: Trauma, Illness and Healing in a Toxic Culture* (Toronto: Vermilion, 2022).

The development of the capacity for feeling, physical pain and emotions alike, is a biological adaptive mechanism meant to enhance chances of survival amidst threats to survival. Pain tells an organism when it needs to remove itself from a setting, situation, or stimulus that is not beneficial to its life. Pain is an evolutionary technology of the embodied living organism that alerts us to being off course; pain tells an animal how well it is doing at survival. Feelings tell us what the organism needs, that some essential balance needs correcting. Denial of the validity of emotions, self-abandonment, the withholding of empathy from another, and other fear-based forms of repression has its origins in the myth of the separate self and the imposed and now often default mindset of scarcity ("there is not enough—money, food, love, compassion—for *me*").[94] Suppression of fear, anger, and other so-called negative emotions is the precursor to rage, which might be suppressed but never fully contained, festering and finding expression externally, through violence against another, or internally, as self-harm, pain, and disease.[95] Evolutionary biologists teach us that feeling states, especially pain, develop within the sentient organism as a signal that something is off course that needs correcting in order to ensure survival. The Eurasian magpie teaches us that the capacity to see self as distinct from and connected to another is a precursor to empathy.

WHAT CAN'T BE BOUGHT OR FAKED: PRESENCE, BELONGING, ATTUNEMENT, CONNECTION

Solidarity, the antidote to alienation, necessitates that what ails us be located, articulated, comprehended, understood. Consciousness is a component of witnessing, the essential work of healing trauma and hurt that keeps individuals feeling apart from rather than an integral part of the collective. We have to correct the wounds of erasure. The hermeneutic violence that keeps us from knowing, naming, fully

---

94. Dana C. Jack, *Silencing the Self: Women and Depression* (New York: William Morrow Paperbacks, 1993); Gabor Maté, *When the Body Says No: Understanding the Stress-Disease Connection* (Hoboken: Wiley, 2011); Elaine Scarry, *The Body in Pain: The Making and Unmaking of the World* (New York: Oxford University Press, 1987).
95. John E. Sarno, *Healing Back Pain: The Mind-Body Connection* (New York: Warner Books, 1991); Gabor Maté, *When the Body Says No: The Cost of Hidden Stress* (Toronto: Knopf Canada, 2003).

seeing, what it is we are witnessing. Not a collection of anecdotes but new kinds of scatterplots that paint new pictures in fuller dimensions. Evoking Neil Smith's adage—this, and all components of political liberation require spatial access. Presence, belonging, attunement, and connection are felt. They exist in the air between us, in the energy field that comprises the container of relational reality, and anybody can discern when they are or are not present.

Alienation is the central reason for the mass of unprocessed pain, untended hurt, stuck grief, and other difficult feelings that lurk and linger in the shadows, gnawing at our core being and coloring our felt sense and experience of the world in this disordered way of life, the mess that capital's made of us. In order to alchemize our hurts, we need an attuned witness, an other who can be present. This is more than material. Attuned presence cannot be commodified. We can feel when another person is in tune with us, truly present, and when they are not. We can tell, in our body, when we are resonant in the company we keep and when we are not, and the difference is everything. This absence of witnessing, resonance, empathy, and good company keeps us stuck in old and new hurt, the accumulation of which leaves us seeking relief. We're alienated in so many ways it keeps us from knowing even how to name what needs attention. We don't think to conceive of the absence of caring, attuned attention as harm. It is the fishbowl we've been swimming in without another viable possible alternative to imagine or compare.

Attunement—the work of refining our capacity for presence and resonance together—is the antidote to alienation, which is the root cause of so-called addiction. Attunement is the alchemical base ingredient for transmuting the energetic remnants of trauma and stuck fear. It is attuning to the relational field, becoming aware of the energy in the air between us that allows us to become *mycelial*, our nervous systems booting online to the Earth grid, where we've always belonged but have been disconnected from through programming. Programming looks like the lived and inherited lessons of being on the receiving end of coordinated violence against life. It looks like ideologies and other lies in the mind, put there intentionally or not, in the recent, distant, and ancient past for some purpose or another.

STRANGE LOOPS, NEW GROOVES

Far beyond the captured wealth produced by our labor, capital inverts our whole way of understanding life, subsumes our knowing, our organizing, our way of living at every turn to its logic and its insatiable desire for more of itself. Our consumptive needs are exploited. Our desires are demonized, destroyed, and colonized for gain. The settler-colonial society produces immense and unevenly distributed social pain, produces the capacity to make billions selling a tonic to soothe that pain, and then punishes with cages and other types of spatial confinement the segment of people who take refuge in the soothing tonic. Their use is deemed unruly or too public. Their otherwise disorderly ways of being expose the contradictions and stabilizing lies at the unstable core of it all. In being deemed "bad" or "sick" these individuals do an enormous and unrecognized service for the system's ability to maintain.

Inertia is not stasis; it is the propensity to maintain the momentum of a given, inherited pattern, a default programming, a strange loop. Physical evidence of this fact can be seen on both the surface of the Earth and the brain. Repeated acts wear grooves and imprints that make a given motion, a trajectory of things, foretold, even when not consciously intended. "What fires together, wires together," goes an adage of popular neuroscience. The default state of things, over time, becomes automatic. But this is not to be confused with a deterministic, nor a pessimistic, diagnosis. In recent decades, developments in live brain imaging technologies reveal new depths of knowledge about neuroplasticity, the ability of the brain to reorganize itself by forming new neural connections throughout a lifetime.[96] People can heal. Things can change. *"There ain't nothin' beyond hope,"* to quote Jason Molina, balladeer of the post-NAFTA working class.[97]

We can't diagnose the problem of addiction, or understand the opioid epidemic, if we're looking through capitalism's blinders. We have to understand that addiction is a coping mechanism to life lived in a fundamentally denatured, profit-and-plunder driven social disorder.

---

96. Referring to functional magnetic resonance imaging (fMRI) and positron emission tomography (PET scans).

97. Songs: Ohia, "Back on Top," track 7 on *The Magnolia Electric Co.*, Secretly Canadian, 2003. Molina died in 2013 at the age of thirty-nine from alcoholic organ failure. RIP.

The pain of the paradigm is disproportionately offloaded onto vulnerable people, whether through disposition or social position but almost always both. The paradigm, so good at explaining away its inherent crisis problems, gets us to diagnose disparate problems—flawed genes, immorality, poor luck, unavoidable tragedies, or 'human nature.'

Deterministic science and moralism are employed as a legitimation strategy. Natural/inevitable and anomalous/external are two sides of the coin of how determinist modes of explanation are deployed to explain away a crisis that's existence suggests the terms of order must be rewritten. These thought-terminating cliches hobble our capacity to see what is and isn't natural, normal or inevitable. It constrains our imaginaries of what could otherwise be. It teaches us lies about who we are, what we are, where we are, and why. This hasn't happened through a grand conspiracy, but it will take a coordinated effort to dislodge it. The ideological imaginary of racial, colonial capitalism is at work in the way so-called "addicts" are treated: a premise of inferiority with the option of repentance, salvation within the straitjacket of the system, the paradigm that can only survive by keeping us severed from our souls and deeply felt senses. "You're only as sick as your secrets," goes an adage familiarized by Alcoholics Anonymous (AA). Getting free is the task of rooting out the system's sickness from our souls, becoming and belonging again as one with the living Earth.

Catching the beast by its tail means studying—amid rebrands and repositioned official stories—not what changes but what remain the same. It is from this vantage I've learned to identify and name a dominant tactic of the dead but dominant paradigm: changing discourse instead of changing course. This crisis containment strategy seeks to capture critique and cohere the collective conscious around a new saleable story for the maintenance of the status quo, leaving the structurally embedded patterns of harm in place. It is central to neoliberal governance, with its public relations and management of optics, as those in power seek a short-term fix to maintain their legitimacy rather than the disruption involved with open inquiry into the myriad interrelated social crises we survive in.

This strategy of changing discourse rather than changing course was evident all over my investigation of the opioid epidemic—from state, market, and other kinds of institutional formations with entrenched power structures and extractive ways of being, like academia and the nonprofit industrial complex. We will return to this in Chapter 7, "Addiction as an Accumulation Strategy," where I offer an understanding of the production of containment strategies in the the opioid epidemic, for which sales pitches, sloganeering, turning a buck, and keeping up appearances tend to be the guiding motivations for institutional change. To evoke Nina Simone, the *"same ole thing, same damn thing,"* rather than life-giving, radical change that would correct systemic and structurally embedded harms.

In the dead and dying world disorder, it doesn't matter ultimately what team we're drafted to, only that we root for the pile of rubble that is capitalism's ultimate creation. This assures the system can serve, in the final act, the only thing it's got left to sell. This is how the system wants us to understand being 'satisfied.' Cognitive foreclosure, historical erasure, and partitioned consciousness are essential tools of domination that keep the masses fighting each other in endless rounds of imperialist wars, lost without a map. We turn to the inherently crisis-prone and warfare-bound economic system in the next chapter, "Capital is a Fiend."

At David Zysk's memorial service at the Preble Street soup kitchen in early November 2015, a friend who rose to eulogize him introduced himself by saying, "David and I met at an elite prep school in Warren, Maine." The crowd relished the momentary reprieve found in laughter, since we all knew he meant the Maine State Prison. Even after years of powerful advocacy work, Google will tell you first and mostly that David Zysk was a felon who committed armed robbery, an act carried out under the spell of commodity craving and in the cognitive-material-affective landscape of *no hope and no future.* David's memorial card, made by his colleagues and friends at Preble Street, shows him muscle-y and poised in a blue T-shirt, with his Preble Street name tag around his neck. The backside contains an excerpt from his favorite poem, which he had pinned on his cubicle wall, "September 1, 1939" by W.H. Auden, a fever-pitched reflection on an insane world order on the eve of yet another World War:

All I have is a voice
To undo the folded lie,
The romantic lie in the brain
Of the sensual man-in-the-street
And the lie of Authority
Whose buildings grope the sky:
There is no such thing as the State
And no one exists alone;
Hunger allows no choice
To the citizen or the police;
We must love one another or die.

CHAPTER 5

CAPITAL IS A FIEND

Surpluses that cannot be absorbed are devalued, sometimes even physically destroyed.

—David Harvey, "The Geopolitics of Capitalism"

LOCATING THE COLLECTIVE PRESENT

In the quest to repair or avoid future harms embedded in capitalism, it's tempting to be seduced by those who think we can save ourselves through regulatory law, policy change, and patching up what are sold as capitalism's leaks. We can be swayed by personality driven stories that want us to think we can solve capitalism's embedded violence and catastrophe by simply rooting out the bad guys, the amoral, greedy few who—the system wants us to think—are the problem with an other-wise well-functioning way of organizing life. By zooming in and out in spacetime dimensions, examining other scales, we see the thread that connects the urgent present to the plunderous past. We see that capitalism is a version of imperialism, not, as the official story goes, an enlightened, rational, and scientific break from it. We see that this war-extraction-conquest model is applied to everyone and is every-where. How do we come to see the fragments of ruin as part of a greater whole—not as a conspiracy but rather a disordered way of life?

From the fractured sight of the dead but dominant paradigm, the myriad crises of the present appear discrete. What does the opioid epidemic have to do with climate collapse? From the old paradigm, the parallels must seem absurd. But from a new and necessary vantage—what I call *ecosystemic sight*—the threads connecting these urgent crises become visible. As we take in new perspectives, our increased awareness, knowledge, and understanding creates expanded consciousness, a new collective story, new common ground. We become possessed of instincts, insight, and vision to not only reconcile the lay of the land, but to chart our collective way home, to ourselves, each other, and an Earthly life where all life forms live in common.

Time is too short and life on Earth too precious to pretend the current trajectory can be contained. *Things fall apart. The center cannot hold.* We live in revolutionary times. If your thinking mind does not already know this, your nervous system surely does. Visions of collapse, apocalypse, Armageddon, and world war fill our feeds and paint our imaginaries. Few strategies seem poised to deliver the salvation we need as a species and as a planetary organism. Moral indignation cannot save us. Regulation, tweaks to the formulas, piecemeal changes at the margins cannot save us. An infinite proliferation of new indicators, measuring scales, data points, names for things, or technological invention in the old world's image cannot save us. The biggest arsenal of weaponry in the world, the biggest stack of whatever kind of money, the most fortified fortress cannot save any one or collective of us. Choosing a side in the dead but dominant world's warfare spin cycle cannot save us.

If we are to survive the present it will be thanks to our capacity to jump scale, to establish new kinds of collective perception and understanding that create a quantum consciousness capable of deeply relational thinking, seeing, and knowing. What is required of the human being in the present moment is to become ecosystemic; it requires unlearning two-thousand-plus years of a plunderous pedagogy. To become ecosystemic is to decolonize.

We must uncover and unwind the internalized, inherited, ingrained conditioning that it took to produce humanity as subjects who can be ruled, conquered, subdued, coerced, or enticed to act against our own and the collective's interest. We must confront the parts of us, conscious and otherwise, that pursue the dead but dominant paradigm's zero-sum concept of winning. We must instead come to know ourselves as parts to an integral whole and to understand our self interest in the greater context of the whole whose parts we comprise. If we are to solve, resolve, heal, and evolve out of the present morass, we must recover our capacity to see systems, both produced and in nature.

STOPPAGES AND FLOWS

Death from opioids and opiates is most always the result of suppressed respiration. Too much opioid relaxes the nervous system to the point that the involuntary and necessary muscle contractions involved in respiration cannot be executed, causing stoppage in the flow of breath. Indeed, the drugs are known to bring all the body's circulatory systems to stasis, as 111 million Americans learned during the 2016 Super Bowl: "Opioids block pain signals but can also block activity in the bowel." One of the event's big-ticket commercial advertisement spots promoted Movantik, the newly FDA approved drug for the newly branded condition, "opioid-induced constipation."

Movantik's patent owners, AstraZeneca and Daiichi Sankyo, chose the $10 million, one-minute ad spot to debut its new "awareness campaign" for OIC as well as their patented cure.[1] The ad shone a spotlight on the ubiquity of American opioid use for those who were not otherwise aware and had missed its prominence in both President Obama's State of the Union address and the 2016 presidential election cycle. The innovation of Movantik resolves a double bind of the opioid sale-and-consumption revenue stream. The ad suggested that viewers taking opioids should take Movantik, and with the help of Movantik, they could take more opioids too.

The drug circumvents a natural limit to greater consumption. Marx teaches in the *Grundrisse*, "Capital is the endless and limitless drive to go beyond its limiting barrier. Every boundary it confronts it hence necessarily strives to transcend."[2] In this case, AstraZeneca and Daiichi Sankyo stepped up rather publicly to fill a produced need some found rather unpalatable, "to help Americans take more opiates."[3]

1.   Ahiza Garcia, "Super Bowl Drug Ad Spurs Big Backlash," *CNN*, February 11, 2016, https://money.cnn.com/2016/02/11/news/super-bowl-painkiller-constipation-ad/index.html.
2.   Karl Marx, *Grundrisse: Foundations of the Critique of Political Economy*, trans. Martin Nicolaus (Harmondsworth: Penguin Books, 1973), 410.
3.   David Kroll, "OICisDifferent: The Drug Behind The Super Bowl 50 Constipation Ad," *Forbes*, July 28, 2019, https://www.forbes.com/sites/davidkroll/2016/02/09/

Capital is value in motion, Marx teaches. Stoppages in capital's flows result in crises. When it cannot move, it cannot grow, and instead is devalued and destroyed. Lack of growth is the definition of crisis in the capitalist system. Capitalism is inherently crisis-prone due to the embedded contradiction of the system's requirement for capital circulation—*capital must change hands* in order to be realized as profits—versus the tendency within the system for wealth to amass into fewer and fewer hands. This baked-in problem of the capitalist system is referred to as "crises of overaccumulation."[4] Accumulation crises look like chronic un- and underemployment alongside surpluses of capital without attractive investment opportunities, the falling rate of profit, and effective demand problems, where consumers do not have the money to buy the things the system produces.

The mass of accumulated capital seeking profitable investments—and the increased speed at which it circulates—has intensified the frequency and severity of crises in the so-called modern world. Often, the "creative destruction" of war-making provides the necessary capital to get the system out of its slump and back into growth again. This is what John Maynard Keynes observed about the system that encouraged his advocacy of government intervention—namely, deficit spending in times of economic downturn—to mitigate the severity of crises. It is also implicit in what President Dwight Eisenhower observed and cautioned against when he coined the term "military-industrial complex."

CAPITALISM NEEDS A CONSTANT (SPATIAL) FIX

Capitalism is constantly in crisis. The "good times" are brief, often frenzied, often in hindsight characterized as a collective fugue state or drug-fueled sprees. Financial headlines are rife with mentions of the industry's *addiction* to debt-leveraged buybacks, or a *craze* for mortgage-backed securities. The imperative to grow or die and the rewards afforded to those agents of its growth willing to get swept away in the madness turns irrational ways of being into a rationale unto itself.

---

oicisdifferent-the-drug-behind-the-super-bowl-50-constipation-ad/.
4.   David Harvey. "Revolutionary and Counter-Revolutionary Theory in Geography and the Problem of Ghetto Formation," *Antipode* 4, no. 2 (1972): 1–13.

There is no such thing as infinite growth on a finite planet. Liberal and Keynesian strategies to ameliorate capitalism's inherent social harm through regulation and redistribution are insufficient and only prolong the inevitable need to break from the inherently destructive economic model. Regulations incentivize the reward available to those capitalists who most cleverly undermine them. Whole industries and brilliant minds are put to work in a regulated capitalist market figuring out how best to subvert regulation to turn an extra buck. The profit motive fundamentally misaligns human objectives and the objective of compound growth. An important feature of the system's instability rests on questions of valuation, debt-backed expansion, liquidity, and the real base that secures it—in essence, the Earth itself.

Wealth agglomeration and its attendant crisis problems results from the imperative of the profit motive itself. Competition among capitalists leads to the necessity to cut costs; labor costs chief among them. This is achieved in a number of ways, namely through so-called "labor-saving" technological innovation and through other means, such as union-busting; erasure or avoidance of environmental, labor, and banking system regulations; outsourcing to subsidiary firms; and offshoring to places where the costs of production are cheaper. Labor's share of the profits is always the target for cost-saving measures, limiting the ability of working-class people to buy the goods the system produces. This leads to absorption problems, where the system overproduces relative to what can be sold, gumming up the works. This doesn't only create immense waste but foretells of inevitable crises that the system's agents do their best to stave off but never truly resolve.

Crises are "fixed." The devastation machine gets patched up to run another lap around the globe, devouring what and where it can in the name of profit; this is the dead but dominant disorder's notion of progress. The system requires and produces vast unevenness in wealth, opportunity, environment, and life outcomes. Keynesians and "social liberals" believe in the state's role in "regulating out" the worst of these effects, conflating the well-being of capital (its ability to keep flowing because distribution is kept in check) with the well-being of the people and the Earth.

The system is dependent on circulation and exchange, but its own pursuit produces stoppages. This inherent contradiction, Marx and Engels convincingly argued, means that the system contains the seeds of its own destruction. David Harvey furthered our capacity to conceive of the geographic implications of the system's embedded crises with his concept of the "spatial fix": the way in which capital circulation requires territory, at one scale or another, to affix to, transmute and alchemize into realizable gains. In affixing to a given space—a thing, a place, a body, a fictitious symbol such as a unit of carbon— capital inevitably changes that space, reproduces it in its image, for its ever shorter-term aims, which is always the extraction of the maximum amount of profit. This process is what Henri Lefebvre critiqued as the capitalist "production of space"[5] and Neil Smith elaborated as the wholesale "production" of our way of knowing "nature."[6]

Capital must affix itself spatially, and in doing so, it captures and redefines spaces and places at scales ranging from the sub-particulate to the galactic. The climate crisis, the 2008 subprime bubble and burst, the opioid crisis, can all be understood as "rational" according to the logics and spatialized dynamics of capitalist growth. Ever-growing profits must constantly be reinvested, chasing ever-more profits, amidst a landscape of fewer and fewer good and safe bets for growth. This is the truth of market instability that is rarely acknowledged by aspatial economic and financial analyses: as wealth and immiseration accumulate on opposite sides of the scales, capitalists are left with ever-fewer options for absorbing and growing all the world's accumulated assets, or what *This American Life*'s Pulitzer Prize-winning piece in the wake of the 2008 crash called the "Giant Pool of Money."[7]

Bourgeois economists speak of capitalist crises as if they are acts of God, befalling us with no or little warning. Economists rationalize the embedded crises of the system by naturalizing them, with euphemisms like "a correction," or "turns," as natural as the tide, in something called "the business cycle." These obfuscations contribute to our inability to see or name the system's machinations as the one-same cause of so many seemingly desperate present-day crises. Conflated

5.   Henri Lefebvre, *The Production of Space*, trans. Donald Nicholson-Smith (Malden: Wiley-Blackwell, 1992).

6.   Neil Smith "The Production of Nature," in *Future Natural*, ed. George Robertson, Melinda Mash, et al. (London: Routledge, 1996), 35–54; Neil Smith, *Uneven Development: Nature, Capital, and the Production of Space* (Athens: University of Georgia Press, 2008).

7.   "The Giant Pool of Money." *This American Life*, Episode 355, first aired May 9, 2008, updated July 28, 2012, http://www.thisamericanlife.org/radio-archives/episode/355/the-giant-pool-of-money.

with notions of nature, reason or progress, capitalism persists despite mounting evidence of its inherent destructiveness to life on Earth.

LIBERALISM'S FOUNDATIONAL SLIPPAGE

To dislodge the logic of capital from our own consciousness is a huge project precisely because hundreds of years of the disorder are buttressed by an attendant knowledge system, the very infrastructure by which we make meaning. Mostly, I refer to the tradition of European Enlightenment as the origins of the present's working models of everything from philosophy to musical scales to medicine. The Enlightenment tradition explains away its apparent moral and social harms with appeals to nature and human nature, which presume fundamental perversions regarding what a human being is, what life is for, and what counts as progress. Silvia Federici teaches us of the long history of the ideological project to make life something conquerable, and of the "collaboration between philosophy and state terror."[8] Unwinding this is no easy task, but we do have sufficient and growing resources, both in our archives and our instincts.

For example, geographer Neil Smith helped us comprehend how capitalism colonizes our ways of seeing and knowing, following the slippery and muddled way in which its knowledge system deploys the concept of "nature." He shows that the conventional scientific interpretation of nature in Western thought—that nature is external and separate from society—was in itself a produced notion, and that it coexisted in an unchecked contradiction with a conventional acceptance of a universal nature, the belief that "human beings and their social behaviors are every bit as natural as the so-called external aspects of nature."[9] Capitalism is the result of bourgeois revolution, the outcome of a historically specific process of class struggle. Smith notes, echoing Marx, that there is no natural basis for the development of the capitalist mode of production, where accumulation exists for the sake of accumulation.

---

8. Silvia Federici, *Beyond the Periphery of the Skin: Rethinking, Remaking, Reclaiming the Body in Contemporary Capitalism* (Oakland: PM Press/Kairos, 2020), 78.
9. Neil Smith, *Uneven Development: Nature, Capital, and the Production of Space* (Athens: University of Georgia Press, 2008), 11.

Liberal thought was conceived as a revolutionary ideology, against the divine right of kings, but it should never be conflated with a belief in the cause of liberation. Liberalism's notion of freedom is bound up with the unfreedoms that define it, such as private property and a juridical system meant to punish and erase ways of being that do not allow for abstracted and captured social wealth. Liberal freedom, as it emerged, included the freedom to benefit from the wealth afforded by the fact of enslaved human beings rendered commodity-producing inputs of production on stolen land in the Americas.[10] Liberalism's legitimating logic does enormous ideological work in rendering capitalism's inherent social violence as seemingly natural, normal, deserved or otherwise unavoidable. "Liberalism has always been conservative," Smith reminded us.[11]

The prevalence of official lies—historiography as a smokescreen—in place of the dynamic and telling facts of history are evident nowhere more than in the discipline of economics, which was formalized in tandem with the intellectual and political project of liberalism. One of capitalism's great survival tactics is its ability to hide its necessary social violence—to present as simultaneously a natural while highly scientific phenomenon, involving individuated actors making "rational choices" in their best, personal economic interest. This is the mythical *Homo economicus*—whose conjurers include Adam Smith and David Ricardo—which stands in for human being-ness in all mainstream economic theory and popular commentary. *Homo economicus'* aims are conflated with more dynamic and complex human values; for example, to presuppose that human beings' sense of purpose in living is or ought to be the accumulation of a store of abstract wealth.

Capitalism's paradigm requires pain for gain. Immiseration is the other side of abstracted, co-opted, captured social wealth. Economics' flattening and abstraction of spatial considerations erases awareness of this dialectical relationship, as well as concern for distribution considerations (whose pain is whose gain?). This erasure of space conceals the fact that all wealth, whether mediated through a money

---

10. See Robinson, "Capitalism, Slavery and Bourgeois Historiography."
11. Neil Smith, "The Imperial Present: Liberalism has Always been Conservative," *Geopolitics* 13, no. 4 (September 2008): 736–739, https://doi.org/10.1080/14650040802275651.

mechanism or other measure, comes from the Earth and the applied human labor that turns nature's bounty into socially useful abundance.

THE FETISH OF EQUILIBRIUM

Capital takes flight by forcing human consciousness to depart from the real. The principle of "equilibrium" in classical economic modeling makes the case. We are told the system produces abundance, variety, and choice when in fact it produces scarcity, monoculture, and conscription. We are told the system tends toward "equilibrium," when in fact the system throws life out of balance. Unevenness, not equilibrium, is central to how profits are recouped. This is a geographical process.[12]

The "invisible hand" of the market, we are taught to believe, tends toward a steady state, a balanced center. Equilibrium-based models allow for a cognitive erasure of the fact of capitalism's inherent instability and constant—lingering and erupting—states of crisis. This contributes to the paradigm's treatment of crises as aberrations, which allows for a disavowal of the political nature of capitalist crisis and acknowledgement of the social fallout inherent in them.[13]

In proposing that capitalist markets tend toward a harmonious steady state of equilibrium, disruptions, disorder, and crises can be explained away as outliers or glitches, or dislocated onto individual actors who are presented as the cause of the disharmony. The premise that market mechanisms tend toward balance helps throw our collective knowing off course, seeking instead the right combination of price-quantity pairing, pricing pollution, factoring in a pretend cost to imagine the system might reform its inherent incentive to destroy

---

12. Neil Smith, *The Endgame of Globalization* (New York and London: Routledge, 2005); Giovanni Arrighi, *The Long Twentieth Century: Money, Power, and the Origins of Our Times* (London and New York: Verso, 1994); David Harvey, "The 'New' Imperialism: Accumulation by Dispossession," *Socialist Register* 40 (2004), https://socialistregister.com/index.php/srv/article/view/5811; Rosa Luxemburg, *The Accumulation of Capital* (London: Routledge, 2003).
13. This attitude is apparent in every mainstream explanation of the 2008 global financial crisis. The 2019 *Vice* documentary on the crisis, *Panic! The Untold Story of the 2008 Financial Crisis*, with its footage from a ten-year anniversary reunion among the architects of the crisis response, depicts the consensus view that the public owes a debt of gratitude for mitigating a worse fallout.

the Earth. It wrongly suggests we might find a formula for commodi-ty-centric life that could restore wholeness.

Economic modeling and instruction in the classical tradition assumes a reality in which two (or more) variables can be neatly mapped in a linear or logarithmic function on a two-axis graph. Economists deploy a Latin phrase—*ceteris paribus*—to express the axiom "assume all other factors remain unchanged." Assume all other factors except the one being modeled remain equal, which is to say, irrelevant to the question. "Assume perfect information," is another axiom of economic modeling every economics student has heard; assume all actors in the market know the same things, at the same time. Assume that all par-ties have everything they need to know to make a "rational" decision. The contradiction, however, is that imperfect information and uneven access to knowledge are central to how profits are made. The pageantry of equality, opportunity, and efficiency coats every theory and lesson in the discipline of economics, despite enormous countervailing evidence. Thomas Kuhn points to this type of incoherence in describing when paradigms are ripe for overthrowing, and yet the world order persists in capital's image, counting utils and cheering profits and upticks in the GDP, using stock market indices as a barometer of well-being.[14]

Somehow, despite all we know to the contrary, we persist, each of us passively consenting to the ongoing animation of this collective dis-order. The exegesis of lost histories, the collective work of recon-necting the threads that tie the forced-forgotten past to the present, render new constellations for recognizing previously unseen patterns and commonalities: distorted incentives, misplaced metrics, and methodological madness instantiated in the name and likeness of the growth of capitalist profits.

This work of reconnecting the past to the present is most especially urgent and evident in the wake of the ruin imposed by the global neo-liberal *coup d'état*, which furthered capitalist consciousness and tore asunder our cognitive capacity to see and know what is real and true versus what is fake, spin, propaganda, misrepresentation, or otherwise

---

14. Thomas S. Kuhn, *The Structure of Scientific Revolutions* (Chicago: University of Chi-cago Press, 1962); David Harvey, "Revolutionary and Counter Revolutionary Theory in Geography and the Problem of Ghetto Formation," *Antipode* 4, no. 2 (1972), https://doi.org/10.1111/j.1467-8330.1972.tb00486.

a violent lie.[15] The task of uncovering lost histories that beget new and useful theories is essential for helping us adequately see and know our location in the present, embodied, relational here and now. This is the project of producing revolutionary consciousness. The goal is to train our capacity for sight in greater depth and dimension to chart the path to collective liberation.

Entwined with the ideology of liberalism and rooted in a wholesale abstraction from lived time and space, classical economics' two-dimensional paradigm allows for the displacement of capitalism's inherent violence. Liberalism and the liberal version of the myth of the so-called free market is an ordering logic that relies on the isolation of the present from its contexts in space and time. A commodity after all is valuable precisely for its uniformity, its lack of specificity. We still hear the couplet of *free people and free markets* recited like catechism despite all the many contradictions of the present evidence of how capital operates most efficiently in the outright absence of human freedom. Economics distorts that which is observable or instinctual—like an understanding of how collaboration yields results greater than the sum of its parts or that many hands make light work—to render the violence of how capital flows and grows rational, scientific, and irrefutable. Behind the fourth wall of partitioned capitalist consciousness, the so-called invisible hand enacts untold violence, in pursuit of capital's insatiable desire for more, the next fix.

SUPPLY SIDED

Capitalism's inherent crisis problems means its agents are constantly seeking ways to get us on the hook and in on the fix. It not only puts us to work as laborers making more surplus value, but puts us to work circulating and valorizing it, through consumption, willingly or otherwise. Mainstream economics talks about the market as "demand responsive," but the true playbook (in history and the present) reads as follows: create more markets for what you've got to sell; buy cheap; sell dear; make your customer need it for dear life. The discipline of economics and free-market acolytes repeat a refrain: *the market steps up*

---

15. David Harvey, *A Brief History of Neoliberalism* (Oxford: Oxford University Press, 2007).

to fulfill a need. And yet, the world over, we observe a social (dis)order rife with supply-side phenomena, problems introduced precisely by capitalists seeking a market for what they have to sell, producing one by inverting and contorting social need to meet its need for the compound growth of profit.

All of the market-based explanations for fentanyl entering the market, first disguised as or in "heroin," then as its own brand, are all supply-side considerations. Heroin is derived from opium poppies, which are grown in fields in very particular temperate climates. Its cultivation is a process that is subject to the whims of increasingly unpredictable weather patterns, and its harvesting is a labor-intensive process that hasn't yet been mechanized. On the other hand, fentanyl is synthesized in a lab, meaning the inputs can be controlled. Once the initial investment has been made in the lab equipment and brick-and-mortar production facility, very little labor is required in the production process. A desire for higher profit margins, not an insatiable drive for demand on behalf of heroin users but an insatiable desire for more gains from drug-war capitalists, drove the shift from heroin to fentanyl.[16] Through its system of commodity exchange in the service of wealth accumulation, capitalism's slippage in our consciousness allows for a collective conflation of, to paraphrase Ursula K. Le Guin, *goods* with *good.*[17]

HERMENEUTIC VIOLENCE

Smith attributes the taken-for-granted and muddled view of nature in Enlightenment thought as the locus of liberalism's still-present ideological presumption that, "Capitalism is natural; to fight it is to fight human nature."[18] In a denatured world where money mediates exchange, appearances take on a life of their own. The quest for the truth becomes the quest to distinguish the real from the fake, the authentic from the replica, the integral versus the knockoff.

16.   Bryce Pardo et al., "Understanding America's Surge in Fentanyl and Other Synthetic Opioids," October 7, 2019, https://www.rand.org/pubs/research_briefs/RB10091.html.

17.   Ursula K. Le Guin, *The Farthest Shore* (New York: Atheneum, 1972), 258.

18.   Smith, *Uneven Development*, 29.

The story of capitalism is not *survival of the fittest* but survival of the most ruthless and short-sighted. In the competition-driven system, *good* actors are driven out of business by the ones willing to cut corners, subvert regulation, break social contracts, and cause harm. The events that produced the transition to capitalism have been papered over with liberal ideology's narratives of progress, enlightenment, and freedom. Many scholars of the history of capitalism draw our attention to the *ahistoricity* with which the emergence of the system and its state formation(s) is explained.[19] Historian Ellen Meiksins Wood remarks that histories of capitalism are peculiarly nonspecific, and that rather than addressing the compulsory nature of imposition to capitalist social relations, friendly histories speak vaguely and generally of capitalism's origins, as if the turn to market-, money-, and commodity-based ways of being represent a social good or an opportunity rather than a forced conscription.[20]

Capitalist consciousness hobbles our capacity to see commonalities in experience. The project of the expansion of empire is always the project of foreclosing on human consciousness, through acts of enclosure of both the land and our collective knowledge base. Forced forgetting seeks to extinguish the light of consciousness, the torch that illuminates resistance, rebellion and dissent to the encroachment of violence and the imposition of extractive logics.

Forced forgetting is another way to think of the concept of hermeneutic violence. Hermeneutic violence refers to a form of interpretative or communicative violence where there is a distortion, misrepresentation, erasure or oppressive interpretation of a text, idea, culture, or experience. It is a kind of foreclosure in a capacity to know what has been occluded, tampered with, or expunged in a social order's system of knowledge or way of making meaning. In the rampant and ongoing effort to disguise the parasitic system as natural and oriented toward fairness, progress, expansion, and balance, the system's proponents enact the violence of forced forgetting, erasing our collective memory and ways of knowing of a life outside the profit motive's twisted logic. Forced erasure of ways of seeing are and were central to the project of instantiating market, money, and profit-based social relations. Jailing,

---

19. Lefebvre, *The Production of Space*, 23.
20. Ellen Meiksins Wood, *The Origins of Capitalism: A Longer View* (London: Verso, 1999).

stealing, evicting, indebting, murdering, and enslaving human beings, along with intentional obfuscation, assimilation, and miseducation, are central tactics of dominating Earth's bounty in the name of turning the Earth into private property.

OPIUM AND THE MASSES

Stoppages in its flows is how and why capital blows. Thus, the story of the modern world can be periodized into boom-bust-kaboom cycles. Warfare is baked into the thing itself. Like all other kinds of empires, capitalism requires war-making in order to grow. In the context of the forced forgetting required to turn a warfare-centric accumulation model into a supposedly rational way of life, it makes sense that psychoactive drugs are central, not ancillary, commodities in capitalism. Dependency ensures repeat consumption, thus resolving the problem of effective demand and securing the ongoing circulation needed to ensure the return of ever-growing capital gains to their owner. Drugs are secure assets given that demand for them is relatively inelastic, which is an economics term for demand that is resistant to changes in price. Opium in particular is a safe bet for a perpetual return on profit because unlike many commodities, demand for opium and its derivatives grows during wartime. Reflecting on mercantilist imperial interest in opium in the eighteenth century and beyond, Alfred McCoy writes, "Since opium combined the inelastic demand of a basic foodstuff like rice with the high margins of luxuries like cloves or pepper, it was the epoch's ideal trade good."[21] The more calamity, uncertainty, suffering, and disorder is sewn in pursuit of profit and the power to secure gains in perpetuity, the more demand for drugs increases.

Opium's demand throughout modern human history, its desirability in times of war and peace, render it something of a currency. In times of uncertainty, when war and economic crisis threaten to evaporate the value of other kinds of assets, opium's sure demand makes it a safe bet and thus a liquid store of value. Opium derivatives are

---

21. Alfred McCoy, "The Stimulus of Prohibition: A Critical History of the Global Narcotics Trade," in *Dangerous Harvest: Drug Plants and the Transformation of Indigenous Landscapes,* ed. Michael K. Steinberg, Joseph J. Hobbs, Kent Mathewson (Oxford: Oxford University Press, 2004), 34.

used in wartime as tools not only for treating acute physical pain but also as an antidote to a ruptured consciousness. Opioids soothe the embodied and cognitive pain of the afterlife of war and other trauma, and for centuries have been a tonic for coping with an unlivable set of circumstances in an embodied here and now.

Like land, opium and its derivatives are crisis-time assets, safe bets for a store of value. In Thi Bui's 2017 biographical graphic novel about a Vietnamese family, *The Best We Could Do*, the narrator's grandmother keeps her savings stored in hidden balls of raw opium.[22] In the era of departure from the real and short-term, high-yield, capitalism became increasingly more crisis prone. Amidst the flurry of inflated asset-price valuations and blink-of-an-eye algorithmic movements, capitalists also seek to secure a real base, something safe under the sun, a resilient store of wealth should it all go belly up. Currency regimes and reigning orders come and go. But no matter what comes to pass, the morphine molecule will always have value. No matter what destruction to economic means and exchange wartime or upheaval may bring, it also brings the demand for opium.

David Courtwright, historian of drugs and addiction, illustrates that the "Age of Exploration," the fifteenth to seventeenth-century period of European colonial expedition and conquest, marked the introduction of nearly every psychoactive substance in commodity use today.[23] Empire's requisite abstraction of our species from the contexts and convivialities that make us whole and well, is part and parcel to the popularity of commodified coping mechanisms. No matter which end of the equation, colonizer, colonized, labor power (cannon fodder) for the conquest effort—the profanity of colonization is an insult to the core senses of all people. Denial, avoidance, coping, and covering up—these become the human organism's strategies for seeking a return to the feeling state of balance or fleeing to the feeling state of transcendence.

---

22. Thi Bui, *The Best We Could Do: An Illustrated Memoir* (New York: Abrams, 2017).
23. Excluding alcohol, which was already common in Europe before the Middle Ages.

MURDER, FORCE, ANARCHY, AND DEBT[24]

Even before the COVID-19 pandemic struck in 2020, the world economy seemed poised for yet another large-scale event. The system has been running on fumes and fiction since the last "major correction"—the 2008 crisis. Extreme debt-leveraging; unprecedented monetary injections from the central banks in the largest global economies since 2008; the rapid agglomeration of wealth and acquisition of agricultural land, housing, and other real assets by the world's wealthiest; widespread capital hoarding at the largest banks and corporations indicating anticipation of a sharp downturn.

In *Principles for Dealing with the Changing World Order* (2021), billionaire American investor and hedge fund manager Ray Dalio says he learned to be good at anticipating the future by studying the past. In preparing the reader to be a savvy investor in the uncertain present, he focuses on what he calls "big cycles," namely the rise and fall of empires. Steeped in the paradigm, presuming the patterns to be a natural science, a code he's cracked, he advises his readers how to win big in wartime. Seeing the calamity isn't a call to change the system but an opportunity to capitalize on it. This is the vision of winning in the dead but dominant disorder.

Capitalism proports to be about 'value added' yet demonstrates a penchant for asset stripping. Extractivism is a helpful concept that connects the present economic disease to its colonial and imperialist precedents. *Golpe growth* allows us to see that we inhabit, and are being done in by, an economic system where profit is generated by mining life-force itself. The capitalist system is a world war machine. It takes a trained eye to see it, but once taught, it can't be unseen. Revolutionary strategy must focus on teaching how to see what gets occluded in the name of the world dis-order's ongoingness. Training our capacity for quantum sight is the way beyond the master's tools. It is how we retreat to higher ground, the elevated terrain from which we see the game clearly enough to outsmart it, in time. Transcending partitioned sight, the dead but dominant paradigm unravels, not out of morality or ideology, but because it is proven to be at war with life itself.

---

24. Adopted from W. E. B. Du Bois, "War is Murder, Force, Anarchy and Debt," in *Black Reconstruction in America 1860–1880* (New York: Free Press, 1998), 55.

A SUBSTANCE SYNONYMOUS WITH WAR: THE MORPHINE MOLECULE AND IMPERIAL PAIN FOR PROFIT

Opium and its derivatives are a substance that originates as a beautiful flower. Opium's extraction is meant to quell pain, and its impact on human neurochemistry mimics that of a warm, loving, motherly embrace. It is a substance that delivers a temporary sense of safety and soothing amidst a living hell, internal or external, real or perceived. Opioids and opiates are a substance, a commodity, whose spread and favor tracks war-making, domestic and foreign, across the long reach of empire in space and time.[25] The drug is effective at relieving both pain that is produced in the present now moment as well as pain felt in the now moment that originated in an irreconcilable past.

Morphine, the direct antecedent of heroin, was first isolated from opium, the raw substance produced by the opium poppy, in 1804, by German pharmacist and chemist F.W. Serturner, who named the essence after Morpheus, the Greek god of sleep. Thereafter morphine, in pill and hypodermic-injectable forms, became the most popular form of consumption of the drug, replacing wine or juice-based tincture preparations of raw opium.

Heroin's chemical name is diamorphine. It was first derived from the morphine molecule and named by a German chemist working for Bayer laboratories in 1898 for the "heroic," fearless affective state it instilled in the chemist who, as was common in the day, tested the drug by imbibing it. Morphine had become a popular and known-to-be addictive recreational drug, and also, an effective and popular cough suppressant. The intention for the research that discovered heroin was to develop a "nonaddictive" version of morphine that maintained both its mood-uplifting and cough-suppressant properties. Bayer marketed and sold diamorphine as "heroin," a "nonaddictive morphine," from 1898 to 1910.[26] Purdue Pharma of course employed the same market-

---

25.   Homer, *The Odyssey*, trans. Emily Wilson (New York: Norton, 2017); Pierre Belon, "Travels in the Levant: The Observations of Pierre Belon of Le Mans on Many Singularities and Memorable Things Found in Greece, Turkey, Judaea, Egypt, Arabia and Other Foreign Countries" (1553), trans. James Hogarth; Booth, *Opium: A History*; McCoy, *The Politics of Heroin in Southeast Asia*.

26.   Deborah Moore, "Heroin: A Brief History of Unintended Consequences," *Times Union*, August 22, 2014, https://www.timesunion.com/upstate/article/Heroin-A-brief-history-of-unintended-consequences-5705610.php.

ing tactic, touting OxyContin as a nonaddictive opioid treatment. Oxy-Contin as nonaddictive substance is a bit like how carbon trading can save the climate; it is an absurd premise based on flimsy claims in a partitioned paradigm's logic. It is a sales pitch with nothing behind it besides everything the profit motive can muster, which is enough, it is evident, to shape the world in its image. As Margaret Atwood said, "History does not repeat itself, but it rhymes."[27]

Warfare, at one scale or another, is central to how capitalism solves its internal crisis problems. The opiate-war relationship positions the morphine molecule as something like a reserve currency: a "safe bet" in wartime. Dependency-inducing commodities resolve an inherent contradiction within capitalism, *fixing* its imbedded accumulation problems.[28] Following the morphine molecule throughout time presents a clear illustration of the fatal and necessary coupling of the profit motive with social violence.

Courtwright names the "big three" (alcohol, tobacco, caffeine) and "little three" (opium, coca, cannabis) psychoactive substances whose commodification, mass production, circulation, and consumption have been foundational to the creation of global capitalism.[29] These are commodities that induce dependency, that bolster the ongoing circulation of capital by promoting getting human beings on the hook and in on the fix of resolving capital's inherent crises problems. Commodified, consciousness-altering and embodied-state-altering substances soothe the embedded pain and dislocation of the profit motive's social ordering logics. Of the project of European colonization of the world Courtwright says, "With these psychoactive products they paid their bills, bribed and corrupted their native opponents, pacified their workers and soldiers, and stocked their plantations with field hands."[30] This is how the citizens of 1839 Guangzhou became "addicts" en masse. This is how the world we inhabit was made.

---

27. Margaret Atwood, *The Testaments: The Sequel to The Handmaid's Tale* (New York: Nan A. Talese, 2019).

28. Rosa Luxemburg, *The Accumulation of Capital* (New York and London: Routledge, 2003); Karl Marx, *Capital: Volume II*, trans. David Fernbach (London: Penguin Books, 2006), 572.

29. David T. Courtwright, *Dark Paradise* (Cambridge, MA: Harvard University Press, 2009).

30. Paley, *Drug War Capitalism*, 44.

British imperial rule took hold in India through the East India Company's seizure of control of opium cultivation on the subcontinent.[31] The capture of the opium trade and intensification of production, circulation, and profit extraction therefrom was a fundamental growth strategy for the British Raj.[32] The British Crown sought to resolve its accumulation crises (namely a perpetual balance of payments crisis) by producing world-scale commodity consumption schemes based on opium.[33] Indian novelist, anthropologist, and historian Amitav Ghosh recognizes the Indian labor and land that cultivated opium for more than two hundred years as the backbone of British imperialism on the Indian subcontinent. In an 2008 interview with the BBC about his new novel *Sea of Poppies*, Ghosh said that "all the roads lead back to opium." Opium was "the commodity which financed the British Raj in India."[34] British Indian opium cultivation wound down in accordance with the International Opium Conference treaty, ratified at the Hague in January 1912.[35] Ghosh remarks that it is no coincidence that British colonial rule could not outlast the prohibition, coming to an end a little more than twenty years after cessation.

COMMODITY OPIUM: PAIN RELIEF
IN SOCIETIES STRUCTURED BY WARFARE

Capital, in colonizing our notions of life and nature, creates scarcity amidst a pervasive sense of threat. It offers a proliferation of commodities meant to meet our needs, while severing our connections to self, others, and the land—that which we truly need. Markets and money,

---

31.   John F. Richards, "Opium and the British Indian Empire: The Royal Commission of 1895," *Modern Asian Studies* 36, no. 2 (May 2002): 375–420.

32.   Sarah Deming, "The Economic Importance of Indian Opium and Trade with China on Britain's Economy, 1843–1890," Whitman College, *Economic Working Papers* 25 (Spring 2011); J. Y. Wong, *Deadly Dreams: Opium and the Arrow War (1856–1860) in China* (Cambridge: Cambridge University Press, 1998).

33.   "The Report of the Royal Commission on Opium," *British Medical Journal* 1, no. 1789 (April 13, 1895): 836–837.

34.   See interview with Amitav Ghosh, "'Opium Financed British Rule in India,'" *BBC News*, June 23, 2008, http://news.bbc.co.uk/2/hi/south_asia/7460682.stm.

35.   United Nations Treaty Collection, "International Opium Convention, Signed at the Hague on 23 January 1912," United Nations, https://treaties.un.org/Pages/ViewDetailsIV. aspx?src=TREATY&mtdsg_no=VI-2&chapter=6&Temp=mtdsg4&clang=_en.

profit-seeking and inequality, are not unique to capitalism. What is distinct to capitalism, as Marx demonstrates, is the commodity form.

Opium is a capitalist's dream commodity for its inherent properties of being both dependency-inducing and, importantly, requiring ever-increasing quantities to achieve a given effect. The psycho-physiological effect of the drug is an antidote to the internal violence of the system, that which must be disguised, externalized, or explained as anomalous. Focusing investment on dependency-inducing commodities, and ones whose habituation guarantees that demand will grow, is one way that capitalists secure effective demand and thus compound growth.

OPIUM CONSUMPTION IN CHINA

Opium use in Qing Dynasty-era China became more prevalent alongside economic, social, and geographical dislocation. Economic decline, in part due to the ruinous imposition of agricultural policy mandating the planting of foreign-origin commodity crops like maize and sweet potatoes led to lower food yields. Depressed farmer livelihoods produced insufficient earnings and led to a plummeting price of land. In a massive wave of urbanization, destitute farmers moved to the city. In short, it is a familiar story: the glut of available, cheap opium combined with a wave of socio-spatial dislocation in the wake of painful economic reconfiguration in an empire in decline.

It was Dutch-East Indian Traders who first introduced Bengal-grown opium to Chinese consumers, in the early 1700s. Soon after, Chinese farmers began domestic cultivation of the opium poppy as well. The majority of China's supply of opium was obtained by British East-Indian merchants. Records suggest that the origins of British involvement in the East Indian opium trade began with Elizabeth I's ordering, in 1606, British ships to procure Indian opium and return it to England. East Indian opium, the mass cultivation of which was initiated in Benares and Ghazipur, Uttar Pradesh, by the East India Company and other British merchant and mercenary outfits in the seventeenth century, remained the major source of supply for the Chinese market for nearly two hundred years.[36]

In order to curb the growing problem of opium consumption, and in an effort to limit foreign outflows of silver and outside influence, the Qing government banned the import of opium in 1729. However, the international trade in opium not only continued, but it intensified markedly. Drug policy experts refer to this historical trend as "the stimulus of prohibition."[37] When the governor of Canton forbade the sale and imbibing of opium, illegal sale from British smugglers was not only condoned by the British imperial order but encouraged. Britain was increasingly anxious over an ever-growing trade imbalance, having found no sure commodity, aside from opium, to supply to Chinese consumers to offset the heavy transfers of silver from British consumers to Chinese merchants in exchange for tea, silk, porcelain, and spices.

In 1792, George Macartney, "Britain's first ambassador to China," was sent to renegotiate the terms of trade with China. Seeking the "right" to market access, the events showcase the imperial origins of the cause which Marx and Engels, in the *Communist Manifesto*, refer to as "that single, unconscionable Freedom—Free Trade."[38] Writing in his diary en route to China in 1794, Macartney observed:

> The breaking-up of the power of China (no very improbable event) would occasion a complete subversion of the commerce, not only of Asia, but a very sensible change in the other quarters of the world. The industry and the ingenuity of the Chinese would be checked and enfeebled, but they would not be annihilated. Her ports would no longer be barricaded; they would be attempted by all the adventures of all trading nations, who would search every channel, creek, and cranny of China for a market, and for some time be the cause of much rivalry and disorder. Nevertheless, as Great Britain, from the weight of her riches and the genius and spirits of her people, is become the first political, marine, and commercial Power on the globe, it is reasonable to think that she would prove the greatest gainer by

---

36. Luxemburg, *The Accumulation of Capital*, 367.
37. McCoy, "The Stimulus of Prohibition."
38. Helen Henrietta Macartney Robbins and George Macartney, *Our First Ambassador to China: An Account of the Life of George, Earl of Macartney, with Extracts from His Letters, and the Narrative of His Experiences in China, as Told by Himself, 1737–1806* (Cambridge: Cambridge University Press, 2011).

such a revolution as I have alluded to, and rise superior over every competitor.[39]

In response to Chinese restrictions, Britain declared unfair restrictions on free trade. The British ramped up the illegal smuggling of opium into China in order to generate Chinese silver for the treasury. While British merchants dominated the trade, the allure of the sure-fire way to recoup precious silver by selling a substance that sells itself led more American merchants to enter the Chinese opium trade as well.

Warren Delano II, grandfather to Franklin Delano Roosevelt, had a stake in the illicit opium trade in China. His firm Russell and Company sold opium in China in the nineteenth century. About his involvement, he said, "I do not pretend to justify the prosecution of the opium trade in a moral and philanthropic point of view, but as a merchant I insist that it has been a fair, honorable and legitimate trade."[40] Opium consumption patterns in China saw their first precipitous rise in the late 1700s, in part due to the newly fashionable method of smoking. Unlike the pill or tincture ingestion methods, the smoking method lent a sociality, a ritual nature of the act, hence the emergence of the long-popular opium den. Chinese importation of Indian-grown, British opium rose steadily in the late 1700s. By 1800, nearly 5,000 chests of British opium were imported into China.[41] Increased competition among opium importers drove prices down, and lower prices fueled the spread of the drug's popularity. This is one of many parallels to the present opioid crisis. For example, in New England, the flooding and subsequent restriction of OxyContin opened new markets for heroin, and later fentanyl, there. Locally it became the cheapest available high, reportedly even cheaper than malt liquor.[42]

By 1800, many more British opium merchants were participating in the trade with China. The resulting glut of supply, coupled with the price-deflating impacts of increased competition among vendors,

---

39. Macartney Robbins and Macartney, *Our First Ambassador to China*.

40. Paley, *Drug War Capitalism*, 46.

41. Martin Booth, *Opium: A History* (New York: St. Martin's Griffin, 1999).

42. Katharine Q. Seelye, "Heroin in New England, More Abundant and Deadly," *New York Times*, July 18, 2013, sec. U.S., https://www.nytimes.com/2013/07/19/us/heroin-in-new-england-more-abundant-and-deadly.html.

enhanced the commodity's reach and increased its demand. While opium imbibing initially spread as a luxury partaken by civil servants and wealthy people, the declining price, widescale availability, and increased social dislocation and pain that characterized the moment made the substance an attainable and desirable "luxury" among common people.

THE OPIUM WARS

These were the splendid beginnings of 'opening China' to European civilization— by the opium pipe.

—Rosa Luxemburg, *The Accumulation of Capital*, 1913

The Opium Wars highlight the precapitalist imperial formations that animate the present economic dis-order. They were trade wars that erupted into real wars, in the explicit name of the 'right' to market access, rather the right to get Chinese consumers in on the fix of resolving the British Crown's perpetual debt crisis. Like South American-sourced silver, East Indian-sourced opium circulated worldwide. Like silver, opium was the anchor for enormous worldwide financial and banking sector expansion, and both were integral to the prized sixteenth–to–nineteenth century China trade. Both became assets that secured the ballooning financial economy of debt-backed securities and other forms of commercial paper.

It is estimated that by 1838, between four and twelve million Chinese people were habituated consumers of British-sourced opium, including government officials and other high-status members of society. In this context, the balance of trade fully reversed in British favor, effectively draining China of silver. The economic consequences as well as the visible social crisis of mass dependency led to a Qing-regime policy of prohibition in Canton (modern Guangzhou) in 1839.

Special Imperial Commissioner Lin Zexu was charged with ending the British opium trade *by any means necessary*. Included in his strategies was the introduction of capital punishment for traffickers, but he also petitioned Queen Victoria, appealing to her conscience.[43] In June, Zexu ordered approximately three million pounds of opium seized from the Canton ports and destroyed. British merchants demanded swift retribution. When Britain's demand for reversal of the policy was ignored, war began in 1839 and ended in 1842 with British victory and the Treaty of Nanking, which provisioned war reparations, trading rights at 5 percent tariff in Canton, and access to five free-trade zones known as "treaty ports." It was this treaty that formally ceded Hong Kong, to be held as a British colony until the year 2000.

Historian J.Y. Wong argues in his book *Deadly Dreams: Opium and the Arrow War (1856–1860)* that what in British historical context gets called the Second Opium War is more aptly considered a world war, with Great Britain, France, the United States, and Russia all participating in the right to so-called "free trade" with and in China.[44] Wong argues that the fetish of "national" histories allows for muddled understanding of the history of imperialism. The Opium Wars exemplify how the violent busting up and into markets is how "access to new markets" gets secured, and that the "right" to free trade goes hand and hand throughout history with what the British called "gunboat diplomacy." Dependency-inducing commodity consumption, be it opium or oil, is an essential part of this violence by which the compound growth of profits is secured.

HISTORIOGRAPHY, COMMODITY FETISHISM, AND FIENDISH WAYS

The stories of British opium smuggling and subsequent two wars in China over the "right" to a market hardly ever address the structural nature of the economic imperative to wage war or the insistence on the right to make a mass market selling deleterious, dependency-inducing commodities, instead opting for moralistic tales of human folly. One example, the banner on the Opium Wars section of the British National Army Museum webpage, is satisfyingly straightforward: "In 1839 British forces fought a war on behalf of drug traffickers.

---

43. Ssu-yü Teng and John King Fairbank, *China's Response to the West: A Documentary Survey*, 1839–1923 (Cambridge, MA: Harvard University Press, 1979).
44. Wong, *Deadly Dreams*.

The victory they secured opened up the lucrative China trade to British merchants."[45] The US Drug Enforcement Administration (DEA) Museum's website also features text on the Opium Wars: "In order to fund their ever-increasing desire for Chinese produced tea, Britain, through their control of the East India Company, began smuggling Indian opium to China."[46] Both narratives attribute the cause of the war to criminal, immoral actors and individuals with insatiable desire. This fetishization of the commodity takes on an absurdity in the DEA's story, which proposes the willingness to wage *all-out war*, twice, in order to *drink tea*.

Commodity fetishism is an integral trope used to produce the contorted consciousness required for the passive consent to the present state of things. The stories that emerge and are retold are not a conspiracy but are a legitimation strategy, as they act against revolutionary consciousness about needed structural change. We are meant to disparage not the economic logic that governs the turning of our world but the greed of a few, the misguided fiending for a substance, or other articulations of sinful human frailty. It wasn't the appetite for the commodity tea that led to Britain's insistence in selling the only thing for which Chinese consumers would give up precious flecks of South American, African-slave-mined silver. It was the necessity to acquire capital. The viability of the regime, the Crown, the British Empire, rest on its ability to service its debts. The necessity to acquire new sources for the inflow of capital, represented, in this case, as bits of precious metals and numbers in ledgers, was needed to secure the balance of payments. Opium secured the purse. It, along with the capacity wage and win war, was the liquid asset that backed the banking and currency reserves, accounting measures that allowed for leveraged, debt-based spending to secure the one and only thing that matters in such a system: ongoing growth.

---

45. National Army Museum, "The First China War," https://www.nam.ac.uk/explore/first-china-war-1839-1842.
46. "Opium Poppy," Drug Enforcement Administration (DEA) Museum, https://museum.dea.gov/exhibits/online-exhibits/cannabis-coca-and-poppy-natures-addictive-plants/opium-poppy.

MONEY TROUBLE

The end of the Napoleonic Wars in November 1815 was the culmination of more than a century and a half of inter-imperial (Dutch-Anglo followed by Anglo-French) conflict. In 1816, the Bank of England began a massive debt/monetary regime restructuration, consecrated in the massive recoinage program that created standard gold sovereigns and circulating crowns, half-crowns and eventually copper farthings in 1821. The recoinage of silver after a long drought produced a burst of coins. The United Kingdom struck nearly 40 million shillings between 1816 and 1820, 17 million half crowns and 1.3 million silver crowns. In 1821, Great Britain became the first country to formally adopt the gold standard, in which the monetary unit was tied to the value of circulating gold coins. This resulted in the empire minting standardized silver shillings, further reducing the availability of silver for trade in Asia and spurring the British government to press for more trading rights in China. Metal-backed currency regimes are inherently deflationary, limiting the scope of economic growth to the growth of the metallic base that can be unearthed or seized.

Money represents but betrays, Marx says in the *Grundrisse*. Understanding what it betrays, what central distortion and deceit is distilled, compressed, and contained within the money form—whether fiat or bullion—is central to understanding the contradictions at the core of capitalism's explosive and exploitative nature. Money, not unique to capitalist societies, takes on a supra-commodity role in capitalism, imbued with the godlike power to mediate and mete out access to life and death.

The story of the banking and currency conundrum at the heart of the matter in the Opium Wars amounted in its material form to shavings, flecks, coins, and bars of a mined earth mineral—silver—excavated and sourced on stolen, conquered land, by stolen and conquered (enslaved native, South American and captive, commodified, cargoed African) human beings in the Americas. Economists—and many economic historians—too often overlook the need to account for these parts of the history of the world system: that the silver and gold up for grabs in the Canton trade was unearthed by dominated, dehumanized human labor, from a dominated, commodified living Earth, and sourced, the world over, by Spanish and other European traders.

In *My Cocaine Museum*, Michael Taussig describes a visit to the Gold Museum, housed in a bank-owned skyscraper in downtown Bogota:

> To walk through the Gold Museum is to become vaguely conscious of how for millennia the mystery of gold has through myth and stories sustained the basis of money worldwide. But one story is missing. The museum is silent as to the fact that for more than three centuries of Spanish occupation what the colony stood for and depended upon was the labor of slaves from Africa in the gold mines. Indeed, this gold, along with the silver from Mexico and Peru, was what primed the pump of the capitalist take-off in Europe, its *primitive accumulation.*[47]

Exactly one hundred and fifty-five years after Britain's gold-backed global monetary regime began, US President Richard Nixon would end it, unceremoniously decoupling the US dollar—to which the rest of the world's currencies were pegged—from gold, thrusting the world into a hyper-accelerated debt-based monetary world order. In 1971, the year Nixon decoupled the US dollar from gold, he also uttered the wretched phrase *"war on drugs"* for the first time. This launched a new circuit of legitimized, militarized capacity to turn people into money. Yet, licit and illicit drug capitalism is harder to distinguish than ever, and the capital secured from each mingles and mixes in the financial institutions of the world.[48] Dependency-inducing commodities, namely petroleum, were and remain central to securing the present regime, as does the military might that provides assurance for the US Treasury bonds and Federal Reserve banking regime, which upheld the unipolar imperialist world for those residing in the wealthy, seemingly democratic core of the system. The foundations of this world order have been shredded. The alchemical configurations of money,

---

47. Michael T. Taussig, *My Cocaine Museum* (Chicago: University of Chicago Press, 2004), x.
48. Dawn Paley, *Drug War Capitalism* (Oakland: AK Press, 2014); Tom Teodorczuk, "Netflix Documentary Re-Examines HSBC's $881 Million Money-Laundering Scandal," *MarketWatch*, February 24, 2018, https://www.marketwatch.com/story/netflix-documentary-re-examines-hs-bcs-881-million-money-laundering-scandal-2018-02-21; Rajeev Syal, "Drug Money Saved Banks in Global Crisis, Claims UN Advisor," *Observer*, December 13, 2009, sec. World News, https://www.theguardian.com/global/2009/dec/13/drug-money-banks-saved-un-cfief-claims; Louise Story and Stephanie Saul, "Stream of Foreign Wealth Flows to Elite New York Real Estate," *New York Times*, February 7, 2015, sec. New York, https://www.nytimes.com/2015/02/08/nyregion/stream-of-foreign-wealth-flows-to-time-warner-condos.html.

military might, and meaning are being recast amid intensifying out-breaks of worldwide wars for conquest over the terrain of the living Earth and the terrain of our consciousness—what *makes sense*, what we'll stand for.

THE REAL BASE

In its perpetual boom-bust-kaboom cycles, capital in decline promotes a race for *la tierra firma*. Liquid, safe-bet assets, those which can be immediately "realized" or cashed out, are what's needed to secure the system. Connecting the opioid epidemic with climate collapse and the ongoing ramping up of world war allows us to see the fundamental question of the system and its agents' desperate grabs in the present: to keep the capitalist system, which is running on fumes, currently operating on record low reserve margins of real value, afloat. "Nations That Vowed to Halt Global Warming are Expanding Fossil Fuels" announces *The New York Times* on November 8, 2023. The executive director of the UN Environmental Programme (UNEP), Inger Ander-sen, remarked, "The addiction to fossil fuels still has its claws deep in many nations." Sounding like someone observing a loved one with a substance use disorder, she added, "These plans throw humanity's future into question. Governments must stop saying one thing and doing another."[49]

Shame and moral retorts against the agents of extractivism in the present change nothing and distract from the structural logic of the global system on the brink. It's not greed or immorality that motivates this split consciousness; it's the imperatives of compound growth when capital, as it always, inevitably does, runs out of profitable ave-nues and begins to deteriorate. Just like opium needed to be forced on China in two full-blown wars, extractive industry expansion is neces-sary to shore up the banking and financial sector of the present sys-tem. The real asset of the Earth becomes the supreme financial asset, that which backs the loans, insurance contracts and importantly, the

---

49. Fiona Harvey, "'Insanity': Petrostates Planning Huge Expansion of Fossil Fuels, Says UN Report," *The Guardian*, November 8, 2023, https://www.theguardian.com/environment/2023/nov/08/insanity-petrostates-planning-huge-expansion-of-fossil-fuels-says-un-report.

futures market—assets that symbolize the projected future revenues from the expansion. Oil and gas contracts, the right to manufacture and sell weaponry and drugs, the rights to the water and to land, these are what capital's agents seek most to possess. This is why we see rampant expansion in oil and gas mining contracts. These "irrational" decisions, secured through new construction plans to expand, are the only present-day path to quell the global markets—*fear not, fretful herd, more growth is on the way.*

The Opium Wars represent a blueprint for how precapitalist imperial formations become embedded and rendered as the supposed right to ongoing accumulation at any cost. Capitalism is imperialism, which is a state of permanent war. Adequately conceptualizing the present-day opioid crisis requires recovering multidimensional consciousness.

Questions of spatiality are inherently questions of distribution. To speak of capital's location is to speak of who has it. This concept is central to understanding the violence that is foundational to the capitalist system and to the flattened, tautological paradigm of economics. That capitalism is predicated on the singular goal of the compound growth of capital belies another central conceit in eliminating concerns for spatiality. All value comes from human labor applied to the Earth's resources, and there is only one Earth. Infinite and compounding rates of growth, the premise of profit, is an existential contradiction. If spatiality is central to the augmentation of capital, then space, territory for conquest and accumulation, must constantly be acquired, dominated, destroyed, and produced anew for the system to be viable. Conquest, destruction, extraction, and dependency are central to the system which abstractly values the growth of capitalist profits—not in concert with but in contraindication to—the well-being of humans and the rest of Earth's ecosystem.

Capital is addicted to more of itself and in the present world dis-order the rest unfolds from there. Capital's disordered social order was concretized as scientific and enlightened. It was rendered ontological, "first from second nature," through acts of imperial knowledge production and the instantiation of a worldview that colonized our very way of seeing and knowing ourselves—our bodies, minds, and spirits—and as parts to the whole. Capitalism must rupture the fact of our organismic tethers to one another, that humans are creative and that our collective work brings abundance, in order to supplant in our minds the lie that the capitalist mode of production, or its farcical invisible hand, are the external sources of our wealth, for which we must not only pay but to which we must surrender ourselves, our space and time, and all of the rest of life on Earth.

More American lives have been lost to opioid overdoses in each of the last several years than the total loss of American life in the Vietnam, Iraq, and Afghan wars combined. Understanding of the opioid crisis is enhanced multidimensionally when we see it on a historical continuum with other acts of imperialist warfare, where in the name of growing market share, "stability" and profits, capital's agents secure a fix for ongoing compound growth by getting humans on the hook and in on the fix of resolving the system's inherent crisis problems. Addiction secures the necessary effective demand to keep capital flowing and growing. Opium and its derivatives are a pacification strategy and a growth strategy in a world order structured by the painful pursuit of profit.

When the system's inevitable and embedded crises can no longer be hidden, ignored, or explained away as a natural disaster or anomaly, we're sold tabloid-like tales that locate the problem in personally corrupt individuals motivated by greed or immorality. State actors and other agents of the system seek to contain the fallout of crises to ward off legitimacy crises. They do this by containing people, narratives, and information, and by limiting what can be observed. Evidence of the system's embedded problems are moved geographically—they are outsourced, offshored, and incarcerated. Advertising and propaganda are other essential containment strategies. State and market agents produce spin, craft a narrative, create scapegoats, sell "new and improved" versions of the same old thing. The system is just; the problem is a glitch that will be corrected, a loophole that will be regulated, a handful of bad actors who will be punished.

In *War is a Force That Gives Us Meaning*, Chris Hedges likens war to an addiction to drugs.[50] He describes it as a fix for the problem of alienation, anomie, the gnaw of the mundane amidst a sense that things will never be different, better. He describes the seduction of being at or in war the way I've heard many drug-dependent people describe their relationship to their commodity fix—as a way

---

50. Chris Hedges, *War Is a Force That Gives Us Meaning* (New York: PublicAffairs, 2002).

to structure a life and a reason to get up in the morning. Recalling the brain science about dopamine—what some call "the molecule of more"—it is not the consumption that releases dopamine; it is the seeking. It is having an object in one's sights and taking aim at it that releases the reward chemical. War-making and drug consumption provide a sense of belonging and purpose; a reason for being.

CRISIS AND CONSCIOUSNESS

Consciousness is a matter of how we make sense of what we see, as well as how what we (think we) know affects our capacity for sight. I repeat the words of John Berger, mentioned in Chapter 1: "A large part of seeing is about habit and convention."[51] Capitalism, the ongoing renovation on legacies of imperial violence, succeeds in surviving its constantly produced crisis formations because it pervasively supplants its own logics onto our collective ways of knowing and being together. Capitalism has become the air we breathe even as it poisons the air we breathe. This dead but dominant system's staying power owes to the misconception that the system is somehow natural, intelligent, and the inevitable result of something called "progress."

Capital's ascent was and continues to be paved by transforming existing formations of diversified, localized coexistence into a blank slate; a *tabula rasa* that can be partitioned and rationalized. In addition to taming the landscape, the dimensions of our perceptive senses had to be flattened. Complexity had to be erased and continuities had to be severed. Dynamic systems had to be collapsed in our consciousness into linear logics, ones and zeros, a monoculture. We had to stop seeing Earth, our communities, our bodies, as living systems and instead be indoctrinated to see lifeless space and matter, quantifiable in discrete numbers and units, available to be turned into something mon-. etized, privatized, owned.

Capitalism's only intention, its singular governing logic, at the expense of all life-giving sense, is *more profit*. Like anyone who's ever chased their next high can tell you, all other considerations become

---

51.   John Berger, *Ways of Seeing* (New York: Penguin, 1972).

subsumed by this singular, existential, urgent quest. The search for a never-ending *more* becomes the meaning of life itself.

Rendering visible the tentacles of precapitalist imperial formations that animate the present economic dis-order is urgent to configuring social formations and policies that address the root causes of harm. To bring to light and undo this hermeneutic violence, this forced forgetting of other ways of knowing, being and determining value, is to work towards revolutionary consciousness. Capitalism survives by tapping our veins. It must embed itself into our living systems and colonize our ways of life. In taking its ever-growing, ever-deepening cut, it must subsume more of our life force to its logics and coopt the means of life itself. Capital survives by turning what sustains us into money—the Earth, our connectedness to each other and to nature. Our capacity to nurture and value care, to revere the source of life itself, is severed. It is fitting, then, that among the most common phrases used to describe an opioid high is a warm, motherly embrace.

Marx and Engels rallied the masses with evidence of the system's terminal nature. Capitalism does indeed contain the seeds of its own destruction. The challenge remains for humans to avoid being destroyed along with it. With a paradigm shift, the unity in our struggle becomes evident. Armed with revolutionary sight and insight, we flip the script.

CHAPTER 6

TRAMPS LIKE US

There are parts of the story that are diffused in my body or holding out in some corner of my mind. They don't fit in a linear exposition because they're everywhere and yet no place. There are parts I don't want to analyze or argue—it's enough just to speak, to tell some stories. I'm going for something beyond understanding; I seek resonance. My body tells me when I've found it.

OLNEY, NORTH PHILADELPHIA

To have been born in Olney, North Philadelphia in 1980 is to say that I was born with white skin in a Black ghetto at the then-richest point in the richest country in the history of the world. In the days of the lame-duck Carter Administration, America at the dawn of Ronald Reagan, on the heels of the Vietnam War and the stagflation shocks, in the former-industrial core amidst the halting gears of American industry and the subsequent feeding of the American working class into the meat grinder of finance capital's extractivist logic. At the time of my birth, my parents were scrambling to figure out how to keep their home; formerly my father's parents' home. They did not succeed. Two months shy of my third birthday, we said goodbye to our neighbors, old and new, who my mother says called me the "mayor of the block" because I was always outside on the outdoor-carpeted porch of our compact rowhouse, greeting passersby, curious about their lives and the ways they seemed similar or different to ours.

My mother and father were the child and grandchild, respectively, of immigrants—Irish and Ottoman Greek by way of Argentina. My four grandparents had sixth-grade educations. My mother and father had high school degrees. My dad inherited our three-bedroom row-house from his parents, who, along with his mother's mother and her older brother, purchased it with a mortgage from the Olney Savings and Loan in the mid-1930s. According to my dad's older brother, Uncle Joe, my grandparents lost their previous house, on a different block of the same street, due to the economic downturn of the Great Depression, and so the financing of this new house was an effort to combine the family's modest and dwindling resources by joining forces with more family members. My dad lived at 224 Sulis Street his whole life. Growing up he shared one of the three bedrooms with his two brothers and his Uncle Dan, a World War II veteran who never married.[1] The other rooms were occupied by my dad's parents and my dad's maternal grandmother. After his brothers left the house—one was drafted to Vietnam and the other joined the Peace Corps to avoid being drafted—and everyone else had died, my dad met my mother at a neighborhood bar. Shortly after, she and her four sons, my brothers, joined him to live there in the year before my birth.

During my dad's tenure, Olney was a predominantly Irish neighborhood. His father was the custodian and maintenance man for Incarnation Catholic Church, where my dad and his two brothers attended grade school, and also an occasional bartender at a local pub. My grandmother worked from home doing calligraphy, wedding invitations mostly, and commercial laundry ironing. Both are piecemeal work, paid by the unit, and commonly done in that era by working-class women who had plenty of other and unwaged work to do at home. Once all three of her children were school-aged, she found nine-to-five clerical work downtown.

My dad's stories of his childhood in Olney were envious to me as a kid growing up in settler-Southwest Florida, which at the time was sparsely inhabited. His childhood in Olney was populated with dozens of friends playing in the streets and kin and close family friends stitching the fabric of daily life. My grandfather apparently purchased

---

1.   I have one photo of my paternal great grandparents, Ulster Catholics, standing with Uncle Dan in his uniform. I regret not knowing more about him.

the first color TV on the block, and the family house on Sulis Street became the neighborhood kids' viewing theater. My dad spoke of festive gatherings for celebrations and holidays, of friends and family dropping by, and many a school night involved (surely alcohol-soaked) Irish folk-song sing-alongs that went into late night.

My father had worked as a unionized baker for a family-owned North Philly-based bakery called Hanscom's Bakery since he graduated from the Catholic vocational high school Mercy Tech in 1960, at the age of seventeen. His coworkers and fellow union members, who were also his friends, were mostly men, a mix of white, Black, and Puerto Rican. He was building a handsome pension, had good benefits, and enough money to pay the bills and enjoy a satisfying array of leisure-time activities. In his "bachelor days," as he liked to reminisce, he bought a new car every two years, held season tickets to his beloved Philadelphia Eagles, and even went on annual vacations (Puerto Rico, San Francisco, the Poconos) with family and friends. I know so much about my dad's youth in Olney because of my dad's habit, throughout my lifetime, of reminiscing and ruminating out loud in my presence, and sometimes while buzzed, the two of us watching primetime TV. I could tell you the names and personal business of long-gone people I've never met and the locations and characteristics of long-closed bars I've never visited. I loved these stories, partly because I craved any opportunity for time with my parents, both of whom worked tirelessly, and because they spoke of a sense of place, community, and love-centered connection that was completely foreign to my own 1980s Florida upbringing. Everything about Philadelphia and those days seemed like a distant and foreign world, one I was sure was better than my own and the dissolution of which my parents never stopped mourning.

THE STOUFFER'S FOOD CORPORATION

Shortly after my birth, Hanscom's Bakery sold out to the Stouffer's Foods Corporation, which had been purchased by the Nestlé Corporation in 1973, two years after the dollar was emancipated from gold and the chrysalis of industrial capital became the butterfly of finance capital, to use Marx's language from Volume II of *Capital*. A dizzying rush of corporate mergers and acquisitions took place in debt- and speculative stock-denominated deals. In accordance with the era's deregulation of financial flows and worker's rights, my dad's union was busted, his pension obliterated, wages cut by about two thirds, and his commute increased by about an hour each way, as he had to drive forty miles outside the city to the emerging suburb of King of Prussia, where the Stouffer's baking plant was located.

Nick Reding's masterful book *Methland* (2010) taught me for the first time the universality of this experience, which I, and I suspect my parents and millions of other blue-collar working people assumed until very recently was their personal tragedy, no less their personal failing. Reding corroborates the two-third pay reduction that meat-packing and other Midwestern industrial workers saw to their pay when the unions went away and the agglomeration of capital left modestly educated people in that region scrambling to make ends meet. When the often-cited statistic is referenced that wages for all American workers have, in the aggregate, stagnated in the post-1970s period, when dollars detached from gold and capital fluttered about trading paper and multiplying, no longer needing tethers to place, rarely does anyone consider that the flattened long-run average is predicated on a precipitous drop which left millions in free fall, with only debt—neoliberalism's version of assistance—to fill the gap.

Property taxes and other bills began accumulating, while declining property values occasioned by explicitly racist blockbusting and fear-mongering real-estate practices, partly induced by the crack epidemic, took its toll. In 1982 my father's best friend of fifteen years, a Black man named Freddy, who had left the neighborhood and mortgaged a new house in the New Jersey suburbs just before the dismantling of their livelihoods, committed suicide. Of all the difficult stories my father shared with me over the years, I didn't learn this one until I was thirty-seven; during our last visit together in Florida for Christmas 2017. In October 1983, a flash freeze burst a pipe and there was no money to fix it. And so, with five children, and without running water or heating, my mother called my father's younger brother, the one who survived Vietnam and settled in Florida, Uncle Dan, and packed our suitcases. My parents left their home and the city where they'd made their entire lives for nearly four decades. The family home on Sulis Street was resold at a city auction for $12,000, all of it claimed by debts, to an up-and-coming slumlord who immediately turned it into Section-8 housing. In the wake of so-called urban renewal and in the aftermath of the demolition of 1960s-era public housing blocks in West Philly, the house was quickly occupied by a former project-dwelling family, who were, like the rest of our new neighbors, Black.

Gentrification and ghettoization are two sides of the same coin; both make real-estate capitalists money. The tactics and technology of racialism and racism are conscripted on the built environment and the people making a life in the place capital sets its sights on. Redlining, blockbusting, fearmongering, and rebranding are all intentional tactics deployed to produce differentials in territorially bounded value, the friction between which capital's agents exploit, extract, for profit. People come and go, flee, scamper, or flock; all orchestrated by capital's imperative to stay in motion in order to grow. The phrase "white flight" implies the privilege to choose something better, and surely in many cases, this is true; but the experience of the multiracial, blue-collar working-class is lost in this flattened, binary narrative and losing this thread of common class experience costs us politically.

VENICE, FLORIDA

Venice, Florida is where my Uncle Dan and his family had bought a modest ranch house on a Veteran's Administration loan after he miraculously returned from a year of guerrilla combat, forced by threats of jail by the government of the "Land of the Free" to kill other poor people who believed in the cause of freedom. So, my parents packed up the younger two of my four older brothers and my three-year-old self, and we boarded the Greyhound bus for a forty-hour trip to Venice, to live in the garage at my Uncle Dan's house.

When I was in the worst phase of my nervous system dysregulation and all the various havocs it wreaked on my body, mind, and spirit for the decade beginning around my thirtieth year, when the wheels began falling off the cart of my rational-mind, overachiever, *never-stop* coping mechanisms, I once quipped: how many ACEs (Adverse Childhood Experience "points") is a forty-hour Greyhound bus ride as a three-year-old? The joke was meant to remind me that the lived afterlife of trauma, the embodied terror stored in my being, *made sense*. I had lived my life for decades—until I found the resources, capacity, knowledge, and fellow humans to help me heal it—with the nervous system of a cold and homeless three-year-old.

The town of Venice, Florida was built, named, and incorporated near the very end of the Florida real-estate bubble of the 1920s. For the Brotherhood of Locomotive Engineers, it was a Hail Mary development scheme to rescue the union's about-to-go-bust pension fund. In times of heightened market uncertainty, this is a general rule: land grabs and speculative development intensify, leaving fragile ecosystems more vulnerable than usual to hapless plunder.

The Brotherhood of Locomotive Engineers is a labor union founded in Marshall, Michigan, in May of 1863.[2] It was the first permanent trade organization for railroad workers in the US. The vice president of the union's pension fund, George Webb, oversaw the purchase of thousands of acres of Southwest Florida between the Gulf of Mexico and the Myakka River and hired developer John Nolen to carve the landscape, once the home of the Calusa people and part of the Caloosahatchee cultural region, into a winter resort town and retirement community for the Brotherhood. The real intention was growth for the floundering pension fund in the cutthroat environment of stagnating GDP and low interest on government bonds—the same conundrum that produced the subprime fever that led to the 2008 bust and the whole world found itself in again, until the stimulus of COVID and war.[3] Working with the canal theme that earned the area the name of Venice, houses and other buildings gestured at Northern Italian architectural styles. The development occurred in concert with the extension of the railway from Chicago and other points in the Midwest to Venice, as well as an advertising campaign targeting the Brotherhood and the general public about what a nice place to vacation or retire Venice, Florida would make.

It didn't. The scheme went belly up. With hindsight, the construction of Venice, Florida began after the Florida land boom went bust, which many historians tie to an extremely destructive hurricane that hit South Florida in September 1926. Northern speculators went packing from Florida in droves, and the Brotherhood abandoned the town

---

2. When it was founded, it was known as "the Brotherhood of the Footboard."
3. Robin Harding, "'Japanification' Stalks the US and Europe," *Financial Times*, October 21, 2019, https://www.ft.com/content/43c5d6b8-efe6-11e9-ad1e-4367d8281195.

by the spring of 1928, the year before the Wall Street crash. Venice became a virtual ghost town for years. Webb's nearly 6,000 square-foot mansion, in which he spent only one lavish winter season in 1927, was squatted by "transients" who looted the place, taking even the bathtub.[4] People resumed settling in Venice when the Kentucky Military Institute, a boarding school for boys, bought some of the abandoned buildings for its new campus starting in 1932. More military stimulus ensued. A US Army air base was opened in 1941.

Before I knew anything of planning or the market, the fact that the thriving of human or any other kind of life was an afterthought to the coming-into-being of Venice, Florida was apparent to me; even as a child. The inadvertent developer of what would become the town of Lehigh Acres, Florida, Gerald Gould, is quoted in an article about Florida's speculative real estate history, saying, "We had no concept of people coming to live here. That's the last thing we thought about."[5] Eventually people did come. Between 1980 and 2010, according to the US Census, the population of the State of Florida quadrupled. Many of the new inhabitants were people like us, long-distance economic migrants, people for whom life didn't work anymore where we came from. Pushed from somewhere else more than pulled to the state, where property values were relatively low and wages were abysmally low, kept in check by "right to work" laws, otherwise known as *right to work without a union contract or any reasonable protections, for as little as the capitalists can possibly get away with paying you,* laws.

When my dad's drinking wore out our welcome with Uncle Dan's wife, we moved to a pay-by-the-week motel room within walking distance to the Publix supermarket where my father had found a baking job at the going rate of $3.35 per hour. My mother, who had steady housekeeping and nanny work in Philadelphia, started working at Wendy's, also at minimum wage, with a commute requiring a two-mile walk across a drawbridge over the Intercostal Waterway. She soon picked up nightshift work at the local 24-hour diner called The Clock, across the street from the motel room where the five of us lived.

---

4.   David Hackett, "Historic Home in Venice, Once the BLE's, on Sale for $4 Million," Brotherhood of Locomotive Engineers and Trainmen, October 3, 2003, http://www.ble-t.org/pr/news/headline.asp?id=8024.
5.   Paul Reyes, "Paradise Swamped: The Boom and Bust of the Middle-Class Dream," *Harper's Magazine* (August 2010): 39–48.

In October 1983, the official unemployment rate for the country was 10 percent.[6] Even then, as always in the history of the United States, the skin of the teeth that my family got by on surely could be measured by the whiteness of the skin of our flesh. The unemployment rate in October 1983 for white people with a high school degree was 9 percent, while for Black people with a high school degree, the official unemployment rate was 21.5 percent.

"Uncle Dan, God bless him, gave us the money to get in there," my mom says about our first rental house, after the motel. On a phone call in 2016, I asked my mom for the numbers, and she was lucid enough to give them to me. The rent at the motel was $125 a week. "I was making $2.50 an hour and your dad was making $3.35. That's why I worked every Sunday; I made time and a half." I hear her apologizing, defending herself for not being around. I know she carries this wound, this guilt, of not being able to *do* or *be more*. It shaped so much of how she saw and related to my brothers and me; longing and a feeling of having failed coupled with an indignation of having had to hold so much, of our not really getting what it was like, *the feeling of what happens*, to borrow Antonio Damasio's titular phrase from his book about the body and emotions in the shaping of consciousness.[7] At some point in the late-1980s, Publix stopped paying time and a half on Sundays, but my dad was grandfathered in. At some point in the early 1990s, my dad's cash Christmas bonus, a few hundred dollars and how we had anything under the tree, became a Butterball™ turkey.

With their wages going to feeding their kids and paying their inflated weekly motel rent, eventually my veteran-turned-mailman Uncle Dan helped out with the down payment for the rental of a proper house, which was cheaper per month than the single motel room we all had grown weary of. When my brother Gus turned fourteen, he too started working at Publix and saved up to buy a used Yamaha moped, which became the family's first and only means of transportation until a year later when someone gave us a rusted-out, late-1960s Plymouth with a 4x4 piece of plywood affixed to the place where a rear bumper goes, which cost more in repairs and fines from

---

6.   Bureau of Labor Statistics, Civilian Unemployment Dataset, https://www.bls.gov/charts/employment-situation/civilian-unemployment-rate.htm.
7.   Antonio Damasio, *The Feeling of What Happens: Body and Emotion in the Making of Consciousness* (San Diego: Mariner Books, 2000).

the police (for its extreme deficit of road-readiness) than it was worth. We were giddy with gratitude. On our first day with the car, my mother put my brother Joe and I to work rolling nickels and dimes. As soon as we had enough to afford hot dogs and ice cream cones for everyone, we took a glorious, seat-beltless spin that I'll never forget.[8]

CALOOSAHATCHEE

I grew up acutely aware of the double bind of what Marx called the "doubly freed laborer."[9] Workers under capitalism, as opposed to feudal, indentured or chatteled laborers, were freed in the sense that they were not enslaved or "owned." They were considered human beings and not subhuman property or sub-adult subjects, but they also were freed from access to the land, free from being able to cultivate enough food for subsistence on a parcel, free to find their own damn place to sleep when night comes, free to pay their own way to reproduce their bodies and clean clothes for work the next day, free to pay their own doctor bills, and free to pay their own gravedigger. Marx, and the best twentieth-century Marxist historians of capitalism, remind us that the long history of empire has been built and sustained on accumulation and domination through subjugation and violence.[10]

What I observed about this double bind of the doubly freed laborer as a child in the 1980s, was that there was never enough money to go around, nor time in a day to be earning it. All the while the Dow Jones climbed, and we periodically scampered further inland along with the surviving wildlife, chasing cheaper rent as coastal Florida was haplessly plundered, one real estate speculator's wing-and-a-prayer development after another. My parents were kind, generous, wise,

---

8.　I say it was glorious, but that memory—like all my early childhood memories—is tinged with fear and anxiety. I was happy and disquieted at once, a contradictory state I recognize sometimes today on the faces of poor children accompanied by weary, worried parents.

9.　Karl Marx, *Capital: Volume 1: A Critique of Political Economy*, trans. Ben Fowkes (London: Penguin Classics, 1992). See Chapter 6, "The Buying and Selling of Labour Power."

10.　Cedric J. Robinson, "Capitalism, Slavery and Bourgeois Historiography," *History Workshop Journal* 23, no. 1 (March 1, 1987): 122–140; Ellen Meiksins Wood, *The Origin of Capitalism: A Longer View* (London and New York: Verso, 2002); Giovanni Arrighi, *The Long Twentieth Century: Money, Power and Origins of Our Times* (London and New York: Verso, 1994); Clyde Woods, *Development Arrested: The Blues and Plantation Power in the Mississippi Delta* (London and New York: Verso, 2000).

principled, and big-hearted people. They did their best by us and they always did their best by other people.

Sinking ships amidst Ronald Reagan's rising tide, my parents relentlessly hustled to keep us all alive and fed, paycheck to paycheck. They picked up second (and third) jobs, worked graveyard shifts; they labored fifteen-hour days and were forced to take off subsequent days rather than be paid overtime, per the laws of the day. They were rarely around. When my very stressed and exhausted parents weren't working, they were grieving and reeling. It wasn't just that they felt they had left everyone and everything familiar behind in Philadelphia, but also the sense that everyone and everything didn't exist anymore. Blockbusting and white flight meant that the folks they knew had also left, mostly to newly developed communities on former farmland in New Jersey or the far north suburbs of Philadelphia, and between their traumatized state and their work schedules and lack of disposable income, they didn't make many new friends. They fought; they drank; they fought more. They did their best to stay afloat and care for my brothers and I amidst a perceived reality of no hope, no place, and no future. Eventually, there were pills for the pain associated with the damage done to spines, shoulders, knees, and souls.

The air we breathed in our rental houses was tight with the constricting climate of scarcity, fear, anger, and regret. Gus moved out as soon as he could, having dropped out of high school and working full-time at Publix. Joe was old enough to be mobile, on his bike or skateboard, and started practically living at his best friend's house. By age seven, I was home alone quite often. I cooked myself Stouffer's TV dinners in the microwave and kept myself company with real-crime TV—late-1980s primetime sensations like *America's Most Wanted*. I did my homework in front of the TV on commercial breaks and put myself to bed only to also wake myself up, dress myself, and sort-of successfully braid my own hair. I was mindful of the clock, by which I set out on my banana-seat bicycle, riding through newly bulldozed pine forest, holding my breath hoping to avoid snakes and other scampering wildlife, to arrive at school in the morning.

VIETNAM

I remember Uncle Dan couldn't stand to hear a helicopter. His tour in Vietnam was during the Tet Offensive. He went out on a patrol one day with a few other guys from his unit, and while they were gone their camp was ambushed and the whole unit was wiped out. They came back to camp to find everyone killed.

Uncle Dan came home from the war and stuffed his trunk in the attic at the family home at 224 Sulis Street in Philly. When my parents lost the house, and we took the bus to live in Uncle Dan's garage, it didn't make the move with us, but my brother Michael, who stayed behind in Philly, hung on to it and brought it down one trip in the mid-1980s. After some years in a veteran's support group and walking the hard road to sobriety, Uncle Dan felt up to opening the trunk in 1988 and got the film he found there developed. He shared the photos with me in our rental house on Short Road in Venice. Some of them were of young men drinking, smoking, and goofing around. Others, the ones that still stick in my mind's eye, were of piles of dead bodies, Viet Cong soldiers, or rather Vietnamese farm boys. In some of them, young American GIs posed in front of the piles with their machine guns, making tough grimaces or performed smiles. I can still remember Uncle Dan, speaking in a gentle voice appropriate for a child of my age, wanting to make sure I knew a truth the pictures tried not to disclose: "Of course, right over here," he said, pointing with his nicotine-stained index finger just outside the white border of the black-and-white photo, "there was a pile just as high of our guys. But we didn't take pictures of them."

Uncle Dan allowed me to take some of the photos to my second-grade classroom's weekly show and tell. I smile as I write, recalling this. Healing is the path of re-membering, walking the road back to one's core self, before or beyond all that happened to produce the feeling states and gene expressions of dis-ease. Retrieving this memory feels like connecting to some essence of who I am. I laugh in recognition of myself and say out loud, "*Hello fellow seven-year-old children, have you heard about this fucked-up thing called the Vietnam War? I thought you should know.*"

OSCAR SCHERER STATE PARK

Throughout my older brother Joe's years of struggle with substances and with the state, I often felt helpless, almost confined myself. He'd be out and doing okay, and then wind up back in jail for things like "lying to the judge" in the week's installment of drug court, or as he calls it, "Gotcha Court."

I'd receive the mail I sent him at the county jail back because it supposedly smelled like perfume (I don't use perfume) or contained glitter (it did not). The indignation of not being able to contact my loved one whom the state has locked in a cage, accused of essentially *being bad*, made me want to breathe fire. It was surely a part of the inferno of rage and fear that made my immune system misfire and attack my otherwise healthy body. It was becoming clear. If I didn't find a healthy way to alchemize it, my trapped rage was gonna kill somebody, and it was looking more and more like it'd be me.

My brother Joe taught me about the ideas of eighteenth-century Swedish theologian Emanuel Swedenborg: that heaven and hell can be produced in our minds. Joe couldn't leave the county that last Christmas I was home, in 2017, so after taking him to the courthouse for his daily piss test—he couldn't legally drive either—we went to find the wild at the Oscar Scherer State Park. Joe can tell me the migratory patterns, mating rituals, identifying markings, and other facts about every variety of bird we encounter. He photographs them. His passions are photography, art history, antiques, world history, and birds. Once when Joe had to explain in Gotcha Court why he had been stopped for trespassing in a gated, golf course compound, he responded, "Your honor, I'm a birdaholic." He had been photographing and observing some place that he and the birds knew was wild, but that a deed somewhere restricted.

The landscape of Sabal palms, live oaks, and Spanish moss used to stretch as far as the eye could see in this part of Sarasota County, but just recently nearly everything was bulldozed except the nature preserve whose boundaries we never considered in what seemed to be a limitless expanse of untamed Florida brush. Now you can see the boundaries clearly. It turns out it's not very big.

We took a road to Oscar Scherer that didn't exist three months prior, straight through what had been a vast, formidable wilderness. And on either side, instead of anything wild, now was patted flat earth and big concrete piping. This is the first phase of a new round of speculative housing development—"Homes starting in the $250ks"— announce the billboards, while the number of people who cannot afford homes rapidly rises, and wages stay stagnant and the avenues for getting by, for making a life, dwindle by the day.

Zygmunt Bauman speaks of the circuits of social control in "consumer society": *seduce, sanitize, repress*.[11] Ruth Wilson Gilmore describes the capitalist state's crisis containment strategy: *individualize, isolate, punish*.[12] My brother Joe wore a pink polo shirt that day in December 2017, having scored it from his last stint in court-ordered rehab "for the indigent" at the Salvation Army. During his time there, he spent his days sifting and sorting through donations for the charity shops and getting preached to about how to be good and not bad by a charismatic leader who was shortly later arraigned on securities fraud charges, part of a growing trend of hucksters making a buck selling the state, insurance companies, and investors on a rehab racket. I had encountered this guy during one of my visits to see Joe at "the Sally," as conscripted residents call the Salvation Army rehab. I went to Sunday service where the leader presided; I just didn't trust the guy. To offer another of my mother's phrases, a Mary X-ism, he was *slicker than shit*.

The scheme to get state money into private investors' pockets in the name of "recovery" represented another in a proliferating circuit of finance-driven fixes churning people for whom there is no work into a revenue stream, valuable for their incapacitation, their designation as social waste, the fact of their idled, confined bodies providing the rationale for the supposed improvement schemes that allow capital to flow and grow. It is one instance of the system's penchant for corporeal, embodied, spatial fixes.

HOUSE ARREST, INC.

This trip home, my brother Joe is mandated to blow into a device called Soberlink, a breathalyzer with GPS tracking and a "selfie" camera that

---

11.   Zygmunt Bauman, *Legislators and Interpreters: On Modernity, Post-Modernity, and Intellectuals* (Cambridge: Polity Press, 1987).
12.   Ruth Wilson Gilmore, *Golden Gulag: Prisons, Surplus, Crisis, and Opposition in Globalizing California* (Berkeley: University of California Press, 2007).

every three hours snaps a photo of the person doing the breathing. It bears mentioning that Joe's problem is with opioids, yet the state mandates what it can. In this case, abstinence from alcohol. It is patrolled by a fee-for-service subscription paid for by those conscripted to use it. I learn that on Christmas Eve, he deliberately blew it off and had a couple of cold ones and "sure enough, my probation officer knocks on the door." I gasp. He's laughing, "Christmas Eve, like six o'clock at night." "Dude, fuck the world," I say. "I know it," he giggles before we drift into silence for a minute.

Shortly after Christmas I call to check in and get my seventy-six-year-old mother. She's upset. She has just returned home from dropping my brother Joe off at work at the beachfront seafood restaurant where, despite his felony record, he was given a "chance" as a busboy, thanks to the fact that the managers are fond of the work performed by my seventy-four-year-old father, who is the restaurant's full-time baker, earning $11 an hour. The phone rings and my mother notes that the Caller ID reads, "House Arrest; Indiana." This is the private corporation House Arrest Services, Inc., who are based in Michigan and who have several contracts with the local County Department of Corrections. She answers and is told by the low-waged employee of an out-of-state private contractor that the database shows that my brother Joe missed a "drop" that morning—a urine test, which he is required to leave four or sometimes five times a week, at random, and as notified by a robocall at 7:00 a.m. each day.

The burden of compliance rests on my senior-citizen parents, who share a car. One has a full-time job and the other takes opioids for chronic pain. The phone call informs the morning routine for the whole household. The caller says that if Joe doesn't "drop" by the time the center closes, at 4:00 p.m., that she will have to send the sheriff to arrest him and take him to jail. My mother explains to the woman on the phone that the drop center opens at the exact hour that Joe is meant to start his shift, and that having waited today until ten minutes passed the hour outside a locked door, they chose to leave and try again after work, lest Joe be fired from his job, where after six months of doing good work as a busser, he is being considered for a promotion to server.

Joe is hopeful about the possibility of becoming a server because unlike bussing tables, he might be able to earn enough to pay off his fines and court fees, totaling over $7,000, which he must do if he is ever to hold a driver's license again. This strategy involves putting himself in an environment wherein alcohol and drug use are pervasive. It is a risky option given that succumbing to the temptation to use will land him back in a county-owned cage. He won't be off work before 4:00 p.m., my mom informs her, but they will go "drop" first thing tomorrow. My mom is panicked, but like always, she is denying having any "negative" feelings at all. She tells me of this exchange in a half yell and in disjointed fragments: "If they get their Irish up, they'll go down there and arrest him!"

MUG SHOTS™

On the local news website, I can scroll through a checkerboard mosaic of faces, photos of people who have been "booked." I can read what each was arrested for along with their full names and dates of birth. This is the "Mug Shots" feature of the website.

The font is dramatic, orange, with sort-of evocative lighting. It's very *Cops* (the TV show). The pictures are of people arrested in the area in the last seventy-two hours. In keeping with the demographics of Southwest Florida, most are white. All appear poor, a presumption based on appearances: weathered skin, poor dental hygiene, and certain hair fashion choices. There's a place for "occupation," but for most people it is left blank. "Homeless" read a few. "Roofing" and "Taco Bell" read two others. Below the picture of Joe—thin-cheeked, with wavy hair down to his shoulders; his lips pursed, with the corners of his mouth raised in his classic "*oh shit*" expression—the text reads: "violation of probation, DUI, and 2 counts of possession of a controlled substance without a prescription."

My parents are required to undergo a credit check and leave a deposit in order to receive phone calls from my brother. My parents would not pass the world's most forgiving (or predatory) credit check. They hand over their Social Security numbers and other personal information to the stranger on the phone. The previous day, Joe had called from jail, but without an account having been set up, the calls were immediately rejected.

The rate to receive my brother's calls is $2.50 per minute. As a result of the failed credit check, my parents are required to leave a deposit in order to receive Joe's calls. The suggested deposit is $400. They leave $100. They are told that the calls will be recorded.

THE GULF OF MEXICO

Once Joe drove us an hour away in his very unreliable car to the local marine biology laboratory to volunteer in the rescue mission of an adolescent pygmy sperm whale that had beached itself. The whale, named Luna for its crescent-shaped tail, had fluid in its lungs, and Mote Marine Laboratory had put out a call for around-the-clock volunteers to physically hold up the whale to keep it from sinking.

Joe was so enthusiastic, and I was grateful he wanted me along. We perched Luna on our knees, two at a time in the tank, and we kept the parts of him that emerged from the water wet with damp towels to keep his skin from cracking. I went just the one day, but Joe went several days. He might have even called off work to spend more time with Luna. We got the call on Christmas that Luna had died. Joe and I cried, but Joe, nineteen then to my thirteen years, cried more.

When we were younger still, Joe and I had rescued baby rabbits after our pet cat left them badly wounded on our doorstep. Joe put them in a shoebox and fed them with a dropper, but days later, someone absentmindedly left the door open and the cat got in and killed them all. Joe buried them at the beach but wanted to be alone when he did.

MY FASCIA

I've been working on this project for a long time, and "writers block" doesn't feel apt to describe what I've dealt with getting it finished. I research, synthesize, and write constantly but have struggled when it comes time to put my work out for others. I have needed to confront a series of wrong lessons I learned early in life that led me to associate drawing attention to myself, in this case writing or speaking up from a place of authority, with impending threat to my physical safety.

When I was packing my things for storage in New York before coming to Sweden I came across a photo of myself right around the time I experienced a big fright. I was seven years old. In the photo I'm wearing thrift-store roller skates with mismatched neon laces and the same smile-masking worried face I'm making in practically every early photo of me. I have a fearful child's eyes, the same eyes I see in my brother Joe's latest mugshot. I'm pictured with my best friend at the time, who died, I heard, in her early thirties. Her mother, probably the closest my mother ever had to a friend in the Florida years, died early too, from pills and pain. We are standing in the middle of the street, a block from the Gulf of Mexico, before realtor rebranding turned this patch of sandy, shrubby earth into a luxury commodity, back when it was dusty roads dotted with humble "cracker shacks" occupied by fixed-income seniors and newly arriving *tramps like us*, and with wild boars in the pinewood forest.

I was always trying to protect my parents. I would learn later that this is a classic imprint of the childhood experience in an addictive family system. The degree of worry, fear, rage, and chaos in our home made it impossible for me to trust their love for me, and between their trauma, their constant working, their stress about making ends meet, and the chronic cycles of self-medicating and outbursts of hellish human emotions, I developed a sense that I should not give them more to worry about, that my speaking up would not be welcome by them, that perhaps it would be the thing that made us all fall apart. I was always expecting that second shoe to drop. It was the thing that my fascia, my psoas muscle, my nervous system, was constantly unconsciously braced against. For decades my body lived hardened, on guard, hypervigilant.

Reduce Psychic Tension. I think of Arthur Sackler's tagline from his award-winning Valium campaign. Like a gasp of fresh air, like sunshine and a cool breeze, like the feeling of not even knowing you had tension in your shoulders until it releases, like a deeper and more natural breath than otherwise thought available, like feeling your body's connection to gravity and to the Earth, like feeling the molecules of the self settle, like being served up a portion of peace.

LEWISTON, MAINE

Gabor Maté, in *In the Realm of the Hungry Ghost*, his work on addiction, says that in his years of seeing patients struggling with substance use disorder he didn't encounter a single woman who had not been sexually abused, and that many male patients had been too. Some well-to-do members of the recovery community (who were also entrepreneurs in the market response to the crisis, opening fee-for-service Suboxone clinics in Lewiston and Portland) bankrolled an event with Maté, whose speaker's fee was $20,000. In Lewiston, most people don't make that in a year.

Maté asked the crowd gathered at the Franco-American Cultural Center, a former Catholic church in the style of a French basilica, to raise our hands if we had ever been sexually abused. My heart raced as I raised my hand with at least half of the rest of the audience. He encouraged us to look around the room to notice the number, percentage, of hands in the room. I am not sure about this tactic for making the point but I wasn't going to leave anyone else hanging; and even though I was fearful, I didn't see the point in hiding from such a truth. Only shame would rationalize keeping my hand down, and I rejected that intellectually even if I hadn't beat the demons of shame from my consciousness yet.

In that sense, I appreciated Maté's provocation to just name it, to see and be seen together and not be in isolation; to take the power out of the shame by ignoring it entirely in the name of what is true, not personal or a secret, but a systemic fact. As one Twelve Step adage goes, *secrets keep us sick*. I can remember my hot cheeks, the mild dissociation so common to me then and to most people who live with C-PTSD and other remnants of trauma, my consciousness seemingly hovering above my head, outside my body. I can picture the faces of people I knew who were present as I followed Maté's instructions and looked around the room. I don't remember whose hands were up but I remember who was there, whose faces I can picture in the crowd. David Zysk is in front of me and to the left, wearing a blue flannel and his Preble Street lanyard.

The World Health Organization estimates that one in three women and girls worldwide experience sexual violence. In his paper "The Aetiology of Hysteria," presented in 1896, Sigmund Freud posited that hysteria, for which opiates were prescribed treatment, was the result of traumatic sexual experiences repressed in the unconscious mind. He proposed that these repressed memories of sexual abuse or disturbance, particularly from childhood, manifested as physical and psychological symptoms in adulthood. However, after so many of his colleagues rejected the insinuation that incest and sexual abuse were common among the upper class (from which Freud's patients hailed), Freud retracted the findings. Instead, he put forth the theory of the Oedipus complex, which reframes such accounts from his patients as fantasy rather than real events.

THE GARAGE

My mom wanted to tell me something the last time I saw her at Christmas in 2017. She wanted to tell me, the first person in her life that she was ever going to tell, about what happened to her. *I want to tell you what happened to me,* she said with sincerity, gripping my hand, so thankful I had come home. This was the first time I had seen her since deciding and declaring more than a year earlier that I didn't intend to have anything to do with her unless she acknowledged a few things and went about engaging with me differently. She was so glad I was giving her another chance. She intended to be brave and speak a deep truth. She wanted me to know why she was the way she was. She wanted to get it off her chest.

Maya Angelou had to overcome a fear of her own voice after her speaking up as a child about having been raped led to her rapist being killed. The experience taught young Angelou that her voice was a lethal weapon and led her to go without speaking a word for years. She would later tell a reporter for *The Washington Post* that while she wrote her account of this experience, *I Know Why the Caged Bird Sings,* "I stayed half drunk in the afternoon and cried all night."[13] She knew she needed to speak it, to purge it, but she couldn't do it sober, and so she didn't.

---

13. Michael O'Sullivan, "The 1970 Review of 'I Know Why the Caged Bird Sings,'" *Washington Post*, May 28, 2014, https://www.washingtonpost.com/news/arts-and-entertainment/wp/2014/05/28/the-1970-review-of-i-know-why-the-caged-bird-sings/.

The patio, where my mother, a smoker, spent most of her days, was no longer operational that Christmas on account of the most recent Category 4 hurricane that blew through a couple months prior. The new smoking lounge was the garage, and so there we sat. The fear my mom felt those days in the garage, the fear that courses through my system now, as I recall the memory in order to write it, is the fear of speaking a truth so big it might get you killed. People who live with early childhood trauma think that speaking the truth will be the death of them, or rather the endless torture of them. The fear is the fear of losing your mind, being physically harmed (again), destroyed. Gabor Maté repeats the refrain: *trauma is not what happened to you, it's what's happening now inside of you as a result of what happened to you.*

The thing about traumatic stress, and the constant state of fear and threat that come with it, is that it's not just about a given event or circumstance, past or present; it is everything. It's an epistemology and an ontology, a framework, a way of seeing and knowing the world and of understanding one's self in relation to the whole. Trauma, and especially developmental trauma characterized not by a singular traumatic event but a generalized atmospheric condition of ever-present threats to survival, produces a consciousness of a fractured and incoherent self—amidst, but dissociated from, a fragmented reality.[14] Singer-songwriter Mary Gauthier, who is open about her long-term recovery process, describes the experience of post-traumatic consciousness as the felt sense of anticipating *imminent annihilation.*

The trip passed without my mother telling me most of what she intended to say, but she did say some things. I spent the days watching her try to muster the courage, getting more and more wasted trying to hold the energy of a truth so big as to speak what she was about to speak, about what happened to her. She would start, but then a benzo potentiator would catch up with her morphine molecules, after which

14. Peter A. Levine and Ann Frederick, *Waking the Tiger: Healing Trauma* (Berkeley: North Atlantic Books, 1997); Laurence Heller and Aline LaPierre, *Healing Developmental Trauma: How Early Trauma Affects Self-Regulation, Self-Image, and the Capacity for Relationship* (Berkeley: North Atlantic Books, 2012); Steven Gold, *Not Trauma Alone: Therapy for Child Abuse Survivors in Family and Social Context* (New York and London: Routledge, 2014); Bessel van der Kolk, *The Body Keeps the Score: Brain, Mind, and Body in the Healing of Trauma* (New York: Penguin Books, 2015); Robert Scaer, *The Body Bears the Burden: Trauma, Dissociation, and Disease* (New York and London: Routledge, 2014); Gabor Maté, *In the Realm of Hungry Ghosts: Close Encounters with Addiction* (Berkeley: North Atlantic Books, 2010); Antonio Damasio, *Self Comes to Mind: Constructing the Conscious Brain* (New York: Pantheon, 2010).

she couldn't find her words anymore because she had to focus on finding her breath.

MY THROAT

Throughout my childhood and early adulthood, I had a recurring dream of needing to scream for help and physically not being able to do so. I'd make the motions and press air through my vocal cords, but nothing would happen. I would wake up gasping, sometimes it'd be accompanied by sleep paralysis, where my mind would wake up but I was unable to move my body. The first time I physically lost my voice when I needed it was when I was twenty-two and giving a presentation on my paper in Professor Rick Coe's Intermediate Macroeconomics class at New College of Florida. My paper was on the Mexican Peso Crisis of 1982. I hadn't yet learned David Harvey's theory of the State-Finance Nexus, but I did piece together the case: that the US government's approach to resolving the crisis, containing the contagion, was to bail out the Wall Street investment banks who had made the risky loans, which they did in order to get the needed compound growth on "petrodollar" investments. I would go on to write my undergraduate thesis on Argentina's Peso Collapse of 2001, which I lived firsthand, arriving in Buenos Aires for a seven-month study abroad in June 2002. I understood the two currency collapses, bank runs, to be related and thought studying Mexico's experience would help me better see the mechanisms at play in Argentina.

Like most occasions, I had done my work thoroughly and I was confident in the research and analysis I was presenting. I had gone deep on the topic of balance of payments crises, fixed versus floating exchange rate regimes and the damned-if-you-do-or-don't position that the fiat, debt-denominated dollar regime put nondominant countries in. I was rigorous about the nuances of the IMF's role, a level of understanding that landed me my job at the World Bank. But somewhere in the middle of the presentation, at the front of the class, reading from a paper in my hand, my voice started first to quiver and then to go out. The paper in my hand shook with my nervous system's ramping-up flight response. I was not ashamed of my work but I realize now that having the full attention of the class tripped some wire in me. Mortal danger was alerted. At New College we received narrative evaluations rather than letter or number grades. I don't remember Professor Coe's precise words about my paper, but they were full of praise, glowing. The last sentence of the evaluation I remember intact: "Annie's presentation, however, was not as strong."

When I started my master's degree in International Trade and Investment Policy at George Washington University, I went to the student health center to speak with a doctor about the phenomenon, which I was worried would happen again. In a policy-oriented program, there would be many presentations. The doctor, a white woman in her sixties, upon learning my family history, bluntly asked me why or how I wasn't as fucked up as the rest of my family. I felt offended out of loyalty to them and fidelity to their struggle, as well as misinterpreted. From my vantage, I practically *was* as fucked up as they were.

I'd be asked a version of this question by nearly every doctor, some bosses, several therapists, and colleagues dozens of times after this. I knew that the appearance of my jumping social class was different from reality. My constant state of tension, frequent dissociated panic, and stress-related health conditions told me this, as did my worsening debt-to-income ratio. I couldn't answer her question as all this welled up in my throat. All I could do was deny her the expected social grace of sharing in her disavowal of my family and withdrawal in distrust from her while choking on the rest. She wrote me a prescription for Xanax—a curious choice, having just heard my immediate family's medical history—and set me loose. "Won't this make me drowsy? I need to be alert to give a presentation," I said, hand on the door. "So, drink a cup of coffee with it," she shrugged. The prescription of thirty pills cost about $2 at the pharmacy with my student health insurance plan.

MY HEART

Eight years later my brother Joe would stand trial in Florida for "trafficking" seven, ten-milligram Xanax tablets, or "Xanny bars" as they're called on the street. He faced a sentence of forty-five years for seven pills for which he didn't have a prescription—each ten-milligram pill garnering its own trafficking charge. The pills were found in the back-seat crevice in his car after a minor traffic accident.

On the morning of his trial I called from Maine, a wreck but trying to hide it, wanting to give him a little love and well wishes, not know-ing what would become of him. I would surely have taken a Xanax if I had any; I most definitely smoked some weed, as this was during a several-year period when I smoked dispensary-grade indica for pain most days, several times a day. In typical fashion, Joe offered a masked joviality, seeking to assure me that all was well, wanting to make me laugh despite the potential outcome. He ended the call the way only he would, "Okay I gotta go, but here's a joke for ya. What do you call Joe in a suit?" My affect couldn't switch into humor; I offered only quiet. "No? Come on, no guess? Okay, fine. *DEFENDANT!*," he cack-led before telling me he loved me and hanging up the phone.

CHAPTER 7

ADDICTION AS AN ACCUMULATION STRATEGY

What's that symbol called—the snake eating its own tail? The ouroboros? It's a lot like that. This system works very well, quite well, for everybody involved—except of course for the people who are addicted.

—A private-pay Suboxone-prescribing doctor,
Portland, Maine, September 2015

Capital cannot abide a boundary. So long as there is a world disorder structured around abstract wealth and profits to be made, every social problem will be subsumed to the pursuit of turning a buck. Every human concern, every life-giving and life-threatening concept, can be turned into an *accumulation strategy* that aligns the consensus of human will behind a given course of action, organizing the flow of labor, institutional capacity, logics, and language to conjure the circulation and growth of capital.

Addiction is an accumulation strategy.[1] The opioid epidemic repeats an observable pattern in which a social crisis is produced in accordance with capital's logics, only for the crisis to become another cause for further exploitation and further profits. Amidst sincere community-led efforts to ameliorate and resolve the crisis of opioid dependence and premature death, state-led, market-led, and state-market–led responses demonstrate efforts to contain, capture, and exploit

---

1.   I am inspired to this conceptualization by the work of my mentors David Harvey ("The Body as an Accumulation Strategy," 1998) and Neil Smith ("Nature as an Accumulation Strategy," 2007).

the problem, rather than resolve it. Uncovering paper trails, following the flow of dollars and discourse, reveals the methods by which state and market actors maintain their own interests in the face of the system's produced and worsening crises. Across sectors, places, scales, and kinds of crises, dollars and discourse shapeshift in the name of securing the state and capital's twinned necessities of legitimacy (meaning, at the very least, passive mass consent to the existing power structures) and growing profit. This is the twinned fix the system can't live without.

Capital flows and grows through our beings at every scale imaginable. One way the system manages critique is to titillate us with tales of people *we* (however defined) are *better than*. Systemic crises become personalized, boiled down to flat narratives, tabloid spreads about people who *should be stopped* or *punished*. When we train our sight to extend beyond the widely circulated and unquestioned dramatizations of corrupt individuals acting from greed and immorality—whether on the consumer side (the so-called addict) or the producer side (the Sacklers, for example)—we can see this system's inherent drive to devour life and thus its ill fit for a living planet and a livable future.

Capitalism cannot be "regulated" into being on the side of life. Band-aid, triage, and patchwork approaches to solving the opioid crisis represent inefficacy at best and window-dressing, advertising, and egregious exploitation in the name of "response," "treatment," and "help" at the worst. This chapter brings to light the commonality of state-capital improvement schemes that seek to recoup critique while churning produced waste into new circuits of accumulation and value production. In mapping response efforts, we see the state's central role in "the market."[2] Governance under capitalism isn't only about the "protection of private property" but about the production of new terrains for capitalism, and about securing (producing) spaces for capital to circulate. In other words, we see the system for what it is: imperialism.

Capital reorganizes itself in pursuit of more profit to escape the inevitability of its terminal crisis of overaccumulation. It renovates, reinvents, and rebrands, but rarely does it reflect and course correct. As is evident in what David Harvey has named the "State-Finance

---

2. The discipline of economics considers them separate, even opposing, entities.

Nexus," the containment and exploitation of the opioid crisis demonstrates how neoliberalism succeeds in bringing the capitalist class closer to achieving its ambitions of becoming the state, while the state pursues its goal of remaining the state.

VIVITROL

In the spring of 2017, I listened to a voicemail from my father while on my commute from Bed-Stuy to Midtown Manhattan for the weekly Center for Place, Culture and Politics seminar. It was a typical message from my father: long-form musings about the family and the state of the world. They always ended with *"Bless yourself! Say your prayers!"* And in this era his last words were invariably *"Fuck Trump!"*

This message is mostly about my brother, Joe. Since the Soberlink-related drug court infraction, he's been reincarcerated in the county jail. "He's getting that shot in the ass now that supposedly changes your brain so you don't have cravings. They're giving it to him because he has insurance this time, but the latest is that his insurance dropped him because he hasn't been at work to have an insurance payment come out of his paycheck in thirty days, so we'll see what happens with all that." I quickly realize the drug my father's talking about. Eerily, the subway car I'm sitting in, the station I'm exiting, and the city busses crossing Manhattan are blanketed in ads for Vivitrol, a patented once-monthly injectable delivery format of a long off-patented drug, naltrexone, manufactured by Dublin, Ireland-based pharma firm Alkermes.

Vivitrol is not a "maintenance drug"; it does not contain an opioid. Instead, the drug, which is also approved and used for alcohol dependency, is an opioid antagonist, meaning it blocks opioid receptors in the brain. Studies on the effectiveness of the formula are few, and many conclude that long-term findings are difficult because patients are more likely to discontinue the protocol than with opioid-containing treatments.[3] Evidence suggests that it may be more dangerous

---

3.   National Institute on Drug Abuse, "The Efficacy of Medications in Opioid Use Disorder," *Medications to Treat Opioid Use Disorder Research Report*, May 2023, https://nida.nih.gov/publications/research-reports/medications-to-treat-opioid-addiction/efficacy-medications-opioid-use-disorder.

than opioid-agonist treatment in that people who do return to opioid use are far more likely to suffer an overdose given that one's system has lost its former tolerance for opioids. Another big difference between Vivitrol and other treatments is that to start using the former, the patient needs to have gone through a complete, often painful withdrawal. As discussed in Chapter 3, painful withdrawals have been shown to promote opioid dependence.

The other medications on the market for opioid dependence, methadone and buprenorphine (Suboxone), are "opioid agonists." They are opioids, but the logic behind their use as a recovery-aid from opioid dependence is in the dosing, meaning they bind just enough to opioid receptors to limit cravings or withdrawal symptoms without inducing a high or posing the risks of street-supplied opioids. Suboxone also contains naloxone, the opioid reversal drug. This formulation is meant to deter users from injecting the preparation. More long-term studies on medication assisted therapy (MAT) with opioid replacement drugs are needed, but there is sufficient evidence to render the approach among the best practices currently available in the arsenal of responses to the present epidemic.

Alkermes has used a moralistic, rather than research-based, appeal to lobby for policies and programs that favor Vivitrol over opioid-agonist drugs. The company's CEO has stated on the record that people who take methadone or Suboxone over Vivitrol "aren't strident about wanting to be drug-free."[4] The Comprehensive Addiction and Recovery Act (CARA) was signed into law on July 22, 2016, and was described by Alkermes executives as "a game changer." The law requires that treatment providers, including private rehabs, county jails, and federal prisons offer or provide referrals for the prescribing of all three varieties of FDA-approved medications. The legislation's cosponsors, Senators Rob Portman (R) of Ohio and Sheldon Whitehouse (D) of Rhode Island, were the top two recipients of campaign contributions from Alkermes in the 2016 election cycle.[5]

Through a massive lobbying and sales effort targeting politicians, police departments, judges and corrections officials, the drug

---

4.   Abby Goodnough and Kate Zernike, "Seizing on Opioid Crisis, a Drug Maker Lobbies Hard," *New York Times*, June 11, 2017, https://www.nytimes.com/2017/06/11/health/vivitrol-drug-opioid-addiction.html.
5.   Goodnough and Zernike, "Seizing on Opioid Crisis, a Drug Maker Lobbies Hard."

expanded its sales and growth by 86 percent between 2015 and 2017. Alkermes spent $19 million in federal lobbying from 2010–2017. The 21st Century Cures Act, signed into law on December 13, 2016, mandates states to direct more resources to medication-assisted therapies. As the debates over abstinence-only versus MAT modalities wage on, Alkermes has exploited the rift to sway states into writing legislation and funding programs that allow only for Vivitrol: "We hope to create a gentle federal breeze to kind of sweep behind us—behind our sales really," a sales executive is quoted saying of the strategy.[6]

In recent years, Alkermes has continued to push Vivitrol as a key component in state-level responses to the opioid crisis, maintaining a narrative that emphasizes a "drug-free" approach over other forms of treatment such as methadone or Suboxone. Since the signing of the Trump Administration's opioid response plan in October 2018, which explicitly mentioned Vivitrol as a preferred treatment for people with opioid dependence incarcerated in federal prisons, the drug's prominence has only grown. This legislation contributed to an increase in Alkermes' stock prices and bolstered the company's influence in shaping opioid treatment policy.

By 2024, Vivitrol's integration into state legislation and court systems has expanded even as Vivitrol remains significantly more expensive than its counterparts, with a single monthly injection priced around $1,100. Several states now require treatment centers to offer Vivitrol as part of their opioid crisis response, with some jurisdictions establishing "Vivitrol courts," where participation in drug court programs hinges on the use of this specific medication. As of this year, more than twenty states have effectively enshrined Vivitrol into their legal frameworks, solidifying its role in the nation's ongoing battle against the opioid epidemic.[7]

The debate over the efficacy and ethics of this approach continues. Opioid replacement therapies aren't a perfect fix. Early on, methadone clinics earned a degree of stigma for profit-seeking behavior. Patients and policy makers saw too many of the privately run clinics as being motivated to keep patients hooked on daily drug treatments rather

---

6. Goodnough and Zernike, "Seizing on Opioid Crisis, a Drug Maker Lobbies Hard."
7. National Treatment Court Resource Center, "Treatment Courts across US States/Territories (2023), https://ntcrc.org/wp-content/uploads/2024/06/2023_NTCRC_Treatment-Court_Count_Table.pdf.

than concerned with helping them recover. "Methadonia" describes the condition and its contradictions: it is a state of being, on "the borderland between high and straight," where former heroin users on methadone maintenance "exist" in perpetuity.[8] The problem was a main inspiration for the Young Lords' occupation of Lincoln Hospital in the Bronx in 1970. They saw heroin-dependent people being turned into another circuit of accumulation and decided to take over the treatment facility and try different, noncommodity-fix-based approaches, in pursuit of meaningful healing. The NADA acupuncture protocol was developed in this setting, as a way to support people quitting heroin and methadone. A nervous system and detoxification support tool targeting five points on the ear, the technique is still widely practiced today by harm reductionists and in community health clinics, and is used for a range of conditions beyond substance use, including anxiety and trauma.

While it is true that Suboxone is misused and traded on the street, it is a far safer alternative to street-supplied dope. Often people switch from street dope to Suboxone when trying to hold a job or establish enough stability to begin the arduous process of seeking limited available social services. Those who buy "Subs" on the street do so because they can't access a prescription. In one of the many backwards regulatory contradictions that persists in the present crisis, states strictly limit the number of Suboxone-prescribed patients a given doctor can see. No such limits existed until very recently on the number of opioid prescriptions a doctor can write.[9] A detailed analysis of the MAT debate extends beyond the scope of the present work, but the best argument in favor of MAT is that it keeps would-be street users alive and stable, and, in Gabor Maté's words, "The possibility of renewal exists so long as life exists."[10]

---

8. *Methadonia*, directed by Michel Negroponte (2005; New York: Blackbridge Productions and HBO Documentary), DVD.
9. National Association of State Alcohol and Drug Abuse Directors (NASADAD), "NASADAD Releases Overview of Buprenorphine Patient Limits," January 31, 2019, https://nasadad.org/2019/01/nasadad-releases-overview-of-buprenorphine-patient-limits/.
10. Gabor Maté, *In the Realm of Hungry Ghosts: Close Encounters with Addiction* (Berkeley: North Atlantic Books, 2010).

CHANGING DISCOURSE, NOT CHANGING COURSE

They Talk; We Die.—Young People in Recovery

The neoliberal myth of the suitability of market-based social provisions buttressed a state policy of abandonment and inaction on the opioid epidemic. Public perception that the War on Drugs had been an abysmal, expensive failure, combined with the majority white demographic, and the fact that it was widely known that the epidemic had largely been medically driven, thwarted state actors' attempts to come up with effective and saleable response strategies. All of this combined with the incoherent understanding of the nature of so-called "addiction" produced difficulty coming up with a salient story for the character of the problem. This stalled policy response, with the result being a trend toward patchworked and punitive kinds of "help" and containment strategies. The response measures demonstrate the neoliberal state solution of cops, cages, and other kinds of confinement as "catch-all" solutions to social problems.[11] "Law Enforcement Assisted Diversion" (LEAD), the Law Enforcement Addiction Advocacy Program (LEAAP), among other kinds of police-department led "recovery" initiatives proliferated.[12] Essentially cops and courthouses supplanted the function of case managers, social workers, and community-based care. "Enforcement," like "development," becomes a logic for supposed improvement amidst what Ruth Wilson Gilmore calls a "changing same."[13] While more socially minded interventions and community-led initiatives have been introduced in the past decade or more, the carceral state continues to grow in the name of the opioid epidemic. The jumbled attempts to justify and rationalize *who gets care and who gets cages* exhibit the fault lines in racial order that structure empire's pageantry of deserving and underserving.

---

11. Ruth Wilson Gilmore and Craig Gilmore, "Beyond Bratton," in *Policing the Planet: Why the Policing Crisis Led to Black Lives Matter*, ed. Jordan T. Camp and Christina Heatherton (London and New York: Verso, 2016); Craig Gilmore, *The Real Cost of Prisons Comix*, ed. Lois Ahrens (Oakland: PM Press, 2008).
12. Ford Foundation, *Seattle's Law Enforcement Assisted Diversion Program* (June 2020), https://www.fordfoundation.org/work/learning/research-reports/seattles-law-enforcement-assisted-diversion-program/.
13. Ruth Wilson Gilmore, "Globalisation and US Prison Growth: From Military Keynesianism to Post-Keynesian Militarism," *Race and Class* 40, no. 2–3 (January 1, 1998): 186–188; James Ferguson, *The Anti-Politics Machine: Development, Depoliticization, and Bureaucratic Power in Lesotho* (Minneapolis: University of Minnesota Press, 1994).

Politicians at every scale of government have responded to the opioid crisis with a proliferation of "task forces." "Task force" is an action-oriented term for a meeting. Different ideological stripes paint different constellations as either about care, or cages, or a jumbled mix of the two. In Maine, Governor Paul LePage's task force was law-and-order oriented and populated mostly by DEA and state police agents. The slightly more liberal-leaning state legislature's taskforce had more of a medical bent and was populated with medical experts and wealthy and socially connected parents of overdosed children presenting the narrative "it isn't *who you'd think*; it's people *like us*." I'm not alone in feeling cynical. One can almost hear the same critique in a February 2017 report in the *Portland Press Herald* by Eric Russell, "Maine Lawmakers Create Another Task Force to Address Opiate Crisis." Russell highlights the preponderance of task forces: "The move comes about nine months after a similar task force, established in the summer of 2015 by Gov. Paul LePage, produced a lengthy report filled with recommendations, some of which have been put into action but many of which have not. The new task force comes just weeks after the State Attorney General's Office announced that 378 people had died from drug overdoses in Maine last year, a 39 percent increase over the previous year. Overdose deaths, driven by heroin and fentanyl mostly, have more than doubled in Maine since 2013."[14]

In the state sector, "treatment" was a rationale used to justify the expansion of the carceral state, amidst foreclosure of state and private services and market-based help. For example, in 2015 Mercy Hospital Detox Center in Portland, Maine closed, citing low reimbursement rates from Medicare and private insurance, while attempting to maintain a Christian-ethics-based mission not to deny treatment to uninsured patients. Soon after, the city shuttered the India Street Public Health Clinic.[15] In this vacuum of state support, sinister arguments for "treatment" renovated Governor LePage's previously stalled effort to expand funding for the Maine State Prison.

---

14.   Eric Russell, "Maine Lawmakers Create Another Task Force to Address Opiate Crisis," *Press Herald*, February 17, 2017, https://www.pressherald.com/2017/02/17/maine-lawmakers-create-another-task-force-to-address-opiate-crisis/.
15.   Joe Lawlor, "Plan to Shut City-Run Health Clinic Alarms Patients, Advocates," *Portland Press Herald*, April 14, 2016, https://www.pressherald.com/2016/04/14/plan-to-shut-city-run-health-clinic-alarms-patients-advocates/.

This expansion logic was used by the governor, even though at a public speaking event in Portland he revealed that he does not believe in the efficacy of treatment at all. "We spent $76 million on treatment in 2014," said LePage in response to questions from the audience. "You can go up to $150 million and you're not going to solve the problem. . . . I think that's a disproportionate share of money spent on trying to treat and the success rate is very low." A person in long-term recovery shouted from the crowd: "Does drug treatment work, Mr. Governor?" "Not with heroin," LePage replied.[16] By way of propping up his determinism and justifying his refusal to mobilize state resources on recovery and evidence-based public health response measures, LePage claimed knowledge of a statistic that "90 percent of heroin users eventually die as a result of their addiction."[17] No available studies corroborate this number.

Even progressive politicians attempted to solve the problem with punitive and carceral interventions. In Maine, then Attorney General and future Governor Janet Mills (D) introduced legislation in 2014 to make opioid pill possession without a prescription a felony charge. LD 1554 sought to make "Oxycodone and the aggregate quantity of pills, capsules, tablets, mixtures or substances equal to or more than 30 milligrams" a Class C felony. Again demonstrating the limits of the political imaginary of the neoliberal, carceral containment model, the stated intention of the criminalization legislation was said to be "to get people into treatment." And while more socially minded interventions were introduced in piecemeal and community-led initiatives in the intervening ten years, the trend of carceral containment strategies continues. A congressional bill currently being debated in the Senate, H.R. 467, the "HALT Fentanyl Act," seeks to increase federal prison sentences for fentanyl possession.

When the Maine legislature passed a bill to make naloxone (brand name Narcan) available at pharmacies without a prescription, Governor LePage vetoed the bill, arguing it represented a moral hazard that encouraged users to keep using. On the subject, the national press reported him saying, "naloxone does not truly save lives; it merely

---

16. Christopher Cousins, "Audience Reacts to LePage's Tough Tone at Portland Town Hall," *Bangor Daily News*, December 9, 2015, http://www.bangordailynews.com/2015/12/08/news/audience-reacts-to-lepages-tough-tone-at-portland-town-hall/.

17. Cousins, "Audience Reacts to LePage's Tough Tone at Portland Town Hall."

extends them until the next overdose."[18] Politicians from other states have proposed legislation to charge repeat overdose survivors for the cost of the medical emergency services, or else to ban naloxone prescriptions from them.[19] Academic economists Jennifer Doleac and Anita Mukherjee published a study in 2018 using regression analysis to "demonstrate" a causal link between naloxone accessibility in the US and an increase in emergency room visits for overdoses.[20] The authors purported that naloxone accessibility *increased abuse*. Making the basic error of conflating correlation with causation, the research belies the trap of a main axiom of the discipline, *ceteris paribus* [assume all else constant]. For this reason, the introduction of fentanyl into the supply chain didn't factor into the conclusions. The flawed research findings became dangerous policy ammunition, such as "broadening naloxone access increased the use of fentanyl."[21] Many politicians latched on to this study to bolster their proposals for punitive policy change.

States and counties innovate circuits of "carceral compassion" for those without the wealth to avoid entrapment by the criminal justice system, including the expansion of drug courts and other means of compulsory abstinence enforced by fee-for-service drug testing or forced, non-evidence-based "rehab" run by the Salvation Army and other "indigent service providers" whose revenue streams rely on state-capital circuits of poverty management.[22]

The seemingly separate missions of "treatment," "punishment," "accountability," and "recovery" mingle and meld in the state-market containment effort. Whether framed as medical, therapeutic, or approached from the purely punitive carceral framework,

---

18.   Benedict Carey, "Naloxone Eases Pain of Heroin Epidemic, but Not Without Consequences," *New York Times*, July 28, 2016, https://www.nytimes.com/2016/07/28/us/naloxone-eases-pain-of-heroin-epidemic-but-not-without-consequences.html.

19.   Cleve Wootson, "One Politician's Solution to the Overdose Problem: Let Addicts Die," *Washington Post*, July 28, 2017, https://www.washingtonpost.com/news/to-your-health/wp/2017/06/28/a-council-members-solution-to-his-ohio-towns-overdose-problem-let-addicts-die/; John Bacon, "Ohio Councilman: After 2 Overdoses, No More EMS," *USA Today*, June 28, 2017, https://www.usatoday.com/story/news/nation/2017/06/28/ohio-councilman-suggests-three-strikes-law-halt-overdose-rescues/434920001/.

20.   Jennifer Doleac and Anita Mukherjee, "The Moral Hazard of Lifesaving Innovations: Naloxone Access, Opioid Abuse, and Crime," *SSRN*, February 20, 2018, https://papers.ssrn.com/sol3/papers.cfm?abstract_id=3135264.

21.   Doleac and Mukherjee, "The Moral Hazard of Lifesaving Innovations"

22.   See Judah Schept, *Progressive Punishment: Job Loss, Jail Growth, and the Neoliberal Logic of Carceral Expansion* (New York: NYU Press, 2015).

"rehabilitation" is a narrative of individual violations and personal failure that yields very high profit margins for contracting service providers.

The first "drug courts," which are "specialized court docket programs that target criminal defendants and offenders, juvenile offenders, and parents with pending child welfare cases who have alcohol and other drug dependency problems"[23] was established in Dade County, Florida in 1989. Former Attorney General Janet Reno, who was Florida State Attorney at the time, is among those who led the effort to devise an alternate plan for managing the overwhelming number of drug-related court cases flooding the system at the height of the crack epidemic.[24] In 1994, there were forty-two drug courts in the US. By 2018 there were over 3,100.[25] Scholars on criminal justice reform have called the drug court trend a "quiet revolution."[26]

The proliferation has created a parallel outside-of-prison carceral system with expensive high-tech devices to measure, track, and monitor the person sentenced. The costs are paid by the conscripted person, and "those unable to pay may be re-incarcerated in a cycle that harkens back to debtor's prison."[27] Some tout the innovation as an improvement over mass incarceration, but its logics allow for the criminal dragnet to expand, imprisoning everyday existence. It also makes the firms who manufacture the related technologies and provide contracted services very wealthy.

The lack of cohesive direction highlights the neoliberal state's identity, and legitimacy, crisis. In September 2016, the first big sum of federal money set to be disbursed to states in the name of the opioid crisis was announced and plans for how to spend it felt almost sinister to those of us close to the emergency. The $600,000 sum coming to Maine, the state's senators announced, would be earmarked for

23. Office of Justice Programs, "Drug Courts," *National Institute of Justice*, https://nij.ojp.gov/topics/courts/drug-courts.

24. James L. Nolan, *Reinventing Justice: The American Drug Court Movement* (Princeton: Princeton University Press, 2003).

25. Physicians for Human Rights, *Drug Courts: A Study on the Impact of Drug Courts on People with Substance Use Disorders* (June 2017), https://phr.org/wp-content/uploads/2017/06/phr_drugcourts_report_singlepages.pdf.

26. Kerwin Kaye, *Enforcing Freedom: Drug Courts, Therapeutic Communities, and the Intimacies of the State* (New York: Columbia University Press, 2019).

27. Maya Schenwar, "Incarcerating America," *openDemocracy*, January 19, 2015, https://www.opendemocracy.net/en/opensecurity/incarcerating-america/.

tracking overdose deaths, for *accumulating data.* Amid the fentanyl-induced spike in deaths, Mercy Hospital's detox facility closing for lack of funding, the City of Portland gutting the public health clinic which housed the needle exchange and harm-reduction services center, impossible waitlists for the remaining detox programs, and effectively no treatment options that were either affordable or evidence-based, the decision was practically haunting.

Maine was one of twelve states to earn the funding. The initiative was called "Enhanced State Opioid Overdose Surveillance," something about *rigorous data for rigorous action.* But the action never actually came, just the fetish of data collection as actionable metrics. In March 2019, a *Washington Post* report details that a few years prior, in Fall 2016, eleven public health experts sent a private letter to President Obama explaining that the fentanyl contagion was producing a far more fatal wave of the crisis, and urged the administration to act, but they didn't. "Despite mounting deaths and warnings, the administration did not take extraordinary measures to confront an extraordinary crisis, experts say."[28]

THE REHAB RACKET

Just like methadone patients in the 1990s created the notion of Methadonia, the liminal space between sober and high where heroin users attempting recovery get stuck on a new drug, as a critique of the money-making logics that beget the endless cycle of "maintaining," opioid-dependent people seeking treatment and possessed of health insurance have created a name for the for-profit rehab industry: the "rehab racket" or the "Florida Shuffle."[29] Between 1986 and 2019, the addiction-treatment industry went from being a $9 billion industry to a more than $50 billion industry. Private residential rehab facilities charge at least $10,000 for a one-month stay and can easily cost double

---

28. Scott Higham, Sari Horwitz, and Katie Zezima, "Obama Officials Failed to Focus as Fentanyl Burned Its Way across America," *Washington Post,* March 13, 2019, https://www.washingtonpost.com/graphics/2019/national/fentanyl-epidemic-obama-administration/.

29. Colton Wooten, "My Years in the Florida Shuffle of Drug Addiction," *New Yorker,* October 14, 2019, https://www.newyorker.com/magazine/2019/10/21/my-years-in-the-florida-shuffle-of-drug-addiction.

this amount or more.[30] Recovery entrepreneurs and hucksters alike began opening rehab facilities and sober homes in order to cash in on the new revenue stream.

The Mental Health Parity Act (MHPA) became United States law in September 1996. The law requires health insurance benefits for mental health-related medical treatment match coverage amounts for all other kinds of (physical) health conditions. Prior to this law, private health insurers were not required to cover mental health care. As a part of the Affordable Care Act's legislative effort in 2008, Congress passed an addendum to the Mental Health Parity Act (the Mental Health Parity and Addiction Equity Act), which defined substance use disorder as a mental health condition.

When the ACA went into law—more precisely, in 2014, when subsidized insurance plans proliferated and Medicare extension laws, for states that passed them, went into effect—health care coverage, inclusive of addiction treatment coverage, was extended to 20 million people who previously had not had any.[31] Adding to the number of formerly insured people who newly gained substance-use treatment benefits under the 2008 legislation, suddenly 64 million Americans obtained the right to care for substance-use disorders.

The 21st Century Cures Act and the Comprehensive Addiction and Recovery Act, both passed in 2016, also incentivized revenue streams in the name of opioid addiction and recovery. The long-over-due extension of health care benefits became a windfall for private actors seeking to cash in on the opioid epidemic on the state's dime. In both the private-pay sector and the state-funded carceral circuits, "treatment" rationales and institutional configurations took shape in capital's image.[32]

Players in the rehab racket quickly learned to maximize insurance payouts and began recruiting patients in dubious ways, advertising not only the conventional trappings—such as equine therapy and arts and crafts—but signup incentives like free iPhones. Despite

30. Wooten, "My Years in the Florida Shuffle of Drug Addiction."
31. Center on Budget and Policy Priorities, "Chart Book: Accomplishments of Affordable Care Act," May 5, 2023, https://www.cbpp.org/research/health/chart-book-accomplishments-of-affordable-care-act.
32. Lev Facher, "Kaleo, Maker of $4,100 Overdose Antidote, to Offer Generic for $178," STAT, December 12, 2018, https://www.statnews.com/2018/12/12/kaleo-evzio-overdose-antidote-generic/.

the existence of a Florida Patient Brokering Act, which originally was written to address the practice in for-profit, residential mental health facilities in the 1980s, recruitment efforts and kickbacks for third-party patient-finders became widespread. Brokers are reportedly earning tens of thousands of dollars a year "by wooing vulnerable addicts for treatment centers that often provide few services and sometimes are run by disreputable operators with no training or expertise in drug treatment."

Ubiquitous twelve-step programs—based on the "Twelve Steps" of Alcoholics Anonymous (AA)—are free to anyone and available in church basements and community centers around the world. Nearly every rehab—spanning from the luxury spa, private-pay facilities to the court-ordered, carceral programs for the "indigent"—is based on this model. For decades, treatment programs and modalities, addiction research and theories, have struggled to advance a program more effective than the twelve steps. This is because resolving the problem of so-called addiction requires not that new services be invented but that society itself fundamentally change. Rehab and treatment philosophies run a wide gamut and competition for clients gives many private facilities an artist retreat or summer-vacation vibe. Equine therapy, song-writing, and other feel-good approaches are among the common tactics deployed in pursuit of clients, because as one rehab director told *The New York Times*: "If we went purely science-based, nobody would come to treatment because it would be boring."[33]

Delray Beach, Florida, once known worldwide as a global capital for rehab treatment centers, became regarded instead as "the relapse capital."[34] A report from WLRN, Miami's public radio station, found that Delray Beach's expenditures on naloxone, used to treat opioid overdoses, rose 13,000 percent between 2013 and 2016. This rise outpaced even the exorbitant price hikes in the drug (further evidence of addiction as an accumulation strategy). Palm Beach County launched a sober homes task force, which in its first years of operation

33. Benedict Carey, "In Rehab, 'Two Warring Factions': Abstinence vs. Medication," *New York Times*, December 29, 2018, https://www.nytimes.com/2018/12/29/health/opioid-rehab-abstinence-medication.html.
34. Lizette Alvarez, "Haven for Recovering Addicts Now Profits From Their Relapses," *New York Times*, June 20, 2017, sec. U.S., https://www.nytimes.com/2017/06/20/us/delray-beach-addiction.html.

led to over 100 arrests, with crimes including widespread charges of human trafficking and sexual violence against female patients.[35] The phenomenon was the plot of the 2021 film *Body Brokers.*

THE LIQUID GOLD RUSH

One of the most lucrative schemes hatched by the for-profit, market-based response effort to the opioid crisis has been the proliferation of new methods of urinalysis. A single hi-tech chromatography test can cost thousands of dollars, compared to the traditional "paper strip tests," which cost only a few dollars. Rationales about the new technology being tamper-proof and testing for a wider spectrum of possibly misused substances rendered them payable by insurance.

The lucrative nature of the new methods led many rehabs in Florida to open their own lab facilities. One such lab, it was revealed in court documents in 2014, was approached by Goldman Sachs investors, who valued it a $32 million enterprise.[36] Some estimates suggest a rehab or sober home could generate $20,000 per month, per patient, in urinalysis tests only. A firm called Mercedes Medical, based in Sarasota, Florida, pitched the prospect of setting up in-house urinalysis labs for treatment centers and sober homes throughout the state, saying, "15 samples per day could yield $800,000 in profit!"[37] A source for a *New York Times* investigation into the urine-testing scheme in Florida rehabs called it "a billion-dollar racket," adding, "in a lot of these places, the patients are basically just there to urinate, and management calls them 'thoroughbreds.'"[38]

This practice became ubiquitous. In Maine, a 2016 recovery walk fundraiser called Help ME Recover was sponsored by urine drug-testing company Burlington Labs, whose main revenue stream is court-ordered drug testing. In October 2016, Burlington Labs was subject to a

---

35. US Department of Justice Press Release, "Owner Sentenced to More than 27 Years in Prison for Multi-Million Dollar Health Care Fraud and Money Laundering Scheme Involving Sober Homes and Alcohol and Drug Addiction Treatment Centers," May 17, 2017, https://www.justice.gov/usao-sdfl/pr/owner-sentenced-more-27-years-prison-multi-million-dollar-health-care-fraud-and-money.
36. Wooten, "My Years in the Florida Shuffle of Drug Addiction."
37. David Segal, "In Pursuit of Liquid Gold," *New York Times*, December 27, 2017, sec. Business, https://www.nytimes.com/interactive/2017/12/27/business/urine-test-cost.html.
38. Segal, "In Pursuit of Liquid Gold."

record $6.75 million fine in Vermont, to settle claims that it defrauded the Vermont Medicaid program by billing for multiple drug tests for a single urine sample.[39] The company subsequently rebranded as Aspenti Health.

EVZIO: INELASTIC DEMAND AND THE PRICE OF A LIFE

A commodity with inelastic demand is something that is necessary regardless of the cost. Opportunists often spike the price of a needed good, simply because they can. In recent years, this has become an explicit growth strategy. The most egregious of all examples has been the surging price of all varieties of insulin.[40] EpiPens and the Evzio naloxone auto-injector are other recent examples. Even the cheapest generic formulation of naloxone shot up from $1.84 for two vials in 2005 to $31.66 by 2014, but this pales in comparison to the cost of Evzio, the privately held Kaléo pharmaceutical company's naloxone auto-injector.

Naloxone, a drug made to counter the effects of an opioid over-dose, had been available in generic formulations since 1995. It comes in several delivery mechanisms, including: the cheapest, glass vials that must be drawn up with syringes; a nasal spray; and Kaléo's prod-uct Evzio, a plastic cartridge about the size of a tape cassette that is an auto-injector. With this device, a user merely holds it against the body while pressing the activation button. The primary benefit of an auto-injector is that it is easier for a layperson to use than a syringe. In 2016, the cost of Evzio quintupled: from an already expensive $937.50 for two doses in January to $4,687.50 in April of the same year.[41] As a comparison, in 2018, Narcan nasal spray (another delivery mechanism for naloxone), was one-thirtieth of the cost of Evzio.

39. April McCullum, "Burlington Drug-Testing Company Renamed Following Fraud Settlement," *Burlington Free Press*, July 10, 2017, http://www.burlingtonfreepress.com/story/news/local/2017/07/10/burlington-drug-testing-company-renamed-after-fraud-settlement/463707001/.

40. Ed Silverman, "Insulin Prices Have Skyrocketed, Putting Drug Makers on the Defensive," *STAT*, April 5, 2016, https://www.statnews.com/pharmalot/2016/04/05/insulin-prices-skyrocketed-putting-drug-makers-defensive/.

41. Christina Caron, "Express Scripts Sues Maker of Overdose Drug, Intensifying Feud," *New York Times*, May 31, 2017, https://www.nytimes.com/2017/05/31/health/express-scripts-sues-maker-of-overdose-drug-intensifying-feud.html.

Independent pharma consultant Todd Smith, who is known for advising firms on their price-gouging strategy for (inelastic) essentials, consulted for Kaléo and proposed the Evzio strategy. Smith is mentioned in a 2018 Senate report on the Evzio price-gouging scandal, which stated that the price increase over an eleven-month period was 600 percent. Kaléo got doctors to do "prior authorizations" for Evzio. The drug was covered by Medicare and Medicaid, and the price increase of Evzio cost the programs more than $142 million in 2018, which of course led conservative politicians to decry the cost, not of the price-gouging firm but of people in need of the life-saving medication.[42] The report further stated that Kaléo's Todd Smith-initiated pricing model planned to "capitalize on the opportunity" of the opioid epidemic.[43]

Evzio was the only FDA-approved auto-injector for naloxone, which meant that when Florida, Ohio, and Louisiana passed laws that required first responders to have such approved drugs at hand, between 2015 and 2017, in practice they wrote a law that required Kaléo's product.[44] Baltimore was among several municipalities that encountered shortage problems when their allocated budgets for the drug "ran out" in the midst of this rampant and deliberate price spike.[45] In Philadelphia, the Office of Health and Human Services stated that the high prices of Evzio "have limited the number of doses that [the local government] and its partner organizations can purchase and distribute," and that the cost spike had hampered the ability to save lives in a city where the death toll from opioid overdoses was three times that of homicides and rising. In rural Pennsylvania, a recovery specialist said that she struggled to afford twenty or twenty-five doses but would buy ten times as many if she could afford them.

42. Bacon, "Ohio Councilman."
43. Rob Portman and Tom Carper, "Combatting the Opioid Crisis: The Price Increase of an Opioid Overdose Reversal Drug and the Cost to the U.S. Health Care System," United States Senate Staff Report, 2019, https://www.hsgac.senate.gov/wp-content/uploads/imo/media/doc/Naloxone%20Report%20Final%20with%20Annex1.pdf.
44. Emily Dreyfuss, "The Price of This Opioid Overdose Drug Jumped From $575 to $4,500," Wired, February 15, 2017, https://www.wired.com/2017/02/575-life-saving-drug-jump-4500-blame-perverse-system/.
45. Steven Christensen, "Opioid Epidemic Puts Strain on Baltimore Budget, Naloxone Availability," Baltimore Post-Examiner, April 19, 2018, https://baltimorepostexaminer.com/opioid-epidemic-puts-strain-baltimore-budget-naloxone-availability/2018/04/19.

During this time, Kaléo managed to get a lot of positive press, partly because they donated a lot of auto-injectors to police departments and other first responders. It was later revealed that the bulk of the donated doses were four months from their expiry date at the time of donation. At the Needle Exchange Program in Portland, we received several boxes of near-expiry auto-injectors. After the big price hike in mid-2017, Kaléo gave away hundreds of thousands of doses, but made a caveat in the delivery information to avoid using it on people who were otherwise eligible to get it through Medicare or private insurance.[46]

Price-gouging is merely one way that firms kept life-saving naloxone out of the public's hands. It was recently discovered that Emergent BioSolutions, manufacturer of Narcan nasal spray, made $1.4 billion in profits on the formula while fighting efforts by public health experts to make the treatment available over the counter at pharmacies.[47] The firm fought competitor generic formulations heavily, lobbied municipalities to write their product by name into legislation, and placed representatives of the firm on various government "task forces," blurring the lines between advocacy and promotion.

EVERGREENING FOR "SAFETY"

Chapter 3 addressed the ubiquitous pharma practice of "evergreening," whereby firms petition the FDA for extensions on patent rights by virtue of some necessary and proprietary "improvement." By November 2017, Purdue had been awarded patent extensions on OxyContin as a result of such maneuvers a total of thirteen times.[48] Evidence of overdose deaths, tampering, and diversion of Oxy began mounting early and the firm certainly was aware of this, yet they waited years

46. Max Blau, "Donations of $4,500 Overdose Antidote Were PR Gold for Drug Maker—but Some Kits Were Close to Expiring," STAT, June 18, 2018, https://www.statnews.com/2018/06/18/kaleo-evzio-donations-near-expiration/.
47. Todd C. Frankel, "How One Company Profited While Delaying Narcan's Drugstore Debut," Washington Post, September 18, 2023, sec. Business, https://www.washingtonpost.com/business/2023/09/18/narcan-over-the-counter-delays-emergent-biosolutions/.
48. Katherine Ellen Foley, "Big Pharma Is Taking Advantage of Patent Law to Keep OxyContin from Ever Dying," Quartz, November 18, 2017, https://qz.com/1125690/big-pharma-is-taking-advantage-of-patent-law-to-keep-OxyContin-from-ever-dying/.

to petition the FDA for new patents on the basis of a social need for a new "tamper-proof" formulation.[49]

Starting in 2010, Purdue replaced the original Oxy formulation in the US but not elsewhere, which produced new smuggling routes, first for the original Oxy formulation, still available in Canada, and eventually for counterfeit pressed pill. Fentanyl contagion in the counterfeit pills coming from this route led to a spike in overdoses in the Midwest in about 2014–2017. It was this supply chain that sourced beloved artist Prince's fatal fentanyl overdose.[50]

Firms not only envelop the public critique of their harmful product to win new patents, but drum up scandals of their own. One example is the British multinational firm Reckitt Benckiser. Its product lines mostly comprise drugstore and household staples like dish detergent, condoms, and hair removal cream, but it also manufactures the popular opioid-replacement therapy drug, Suboxone. In 2009, Reckitt Benckiser lost its US patent for Suboxone tablets, which then comprised 85 percent of the total spending on medication-based opioid dependency treatments in the United States.[51] In an attempt to keep generic manufacturers from gaining rights to manufacture and sell cheaper versions of the drug, Reckitt Benckiser simultaneously developed and sought exclusive FDA approval and patent rights for a new, sublingual, individually wrapped, "child-proof," dissolving film version of the drug while setting out to discredit its original, tablet form as a hazard to children. They funded a tailored study to confirm a predetermined conclusion that Suboxone pills in tablet form, distributed in standard pill bottles, were responsible for children's deaths.

Reckitt Benckiser then hired lobbyists to take their manufactured evidence to lawmakers to "raise awareness" of the dangers and

---

49. Josh Katz, "Purdue Pharma, Maker of OxyContin, Is Sued by 2 More States," *New York Times*, May 29, 2018, https://www.nytimes.com/2018/05/29/health/purdue-opioids-oxycontin.html.

50. Silva, "Prince Died after Taking Counterfeit Vicodin Laced with Fentanyl, Prosecutor Says"; Jessica Contrera, "Prince Might Have Been a Casualty of a Counterfeit Pill Problem Sweeping the Nation," *Washington Post*, August 22, 2016, https://www.washingtonpost.com/news/arts-and-entertainment/wp/2016/08/22/prince-might-have-been-the-victim-of-a-counterfeit-pill-problem-sweeping-the-nation/.

51. Chris McGreal, "Reckitt Benckiser Sued by 35 US States for 'profiteering' from Opioid Treatment," *Guardian*, October 21, 2016, sec. Business, https://www.theguardian.com/business/2016/oct/21/reckitt-benckiser-drug-company-sued-suboxone-profiteering-opiod-addiction.

encourage new legislation to mandate purchase of the "tamper proof" films as a matter of public safety.[52] They also raised the price of the tablets to get more of the market to switch to the new film version in advance of any generic competition to the pill form.[53] The FDA did not accept the study as scientifically sound and reported Reckitt Benckiser to the Federal Trade Commission.[54] The case eventually resulted in a $1.4 billion settlement with the US Department of Justice in 2019.

CRISIS, CONTAINMENT, CASHING IN

The jumbled rationales and solutions put in place to respond to the crisis actually serve to fix the state and capital's crises of legitimacy and profitability. A society in capital's image produces untold human suffering and is not equipped with the incentives or institutional configurations to effectively resolve the produced harm. Defeating capitalism requires that we be nimble in tracking its movements and mutations. In particular, we must become more sophisticated in diagnosing the evolving and contradictory ideological, organizational, and material (re)configurations the state uses to put capitalist surpluses *to work*, to render new terrain for capital absorption and valorization, and provide discursive and material conditions for social consent for the machine to go on as it does. Among its ingenious and insidious survival strategies, capital's agents devise ways not only to turn waste into value, but to produce people, places, and things as waste, in order that it might then claim to be solving problems it created. It gets the ever-growing millions of dispossessed, discarded, and otherwise abandoned people and places it produces *on the hook and in on the fix* of resolving its

---

52. McGreal, "Reckitt Benckiser Sued by 35 US States for 'profiteering' from Opioid Treatment"; Youn, "Suboxone Maker Reckitt Benckiser to Pay $1.4 Billion in Largest Opioid Settlement in US History."
53. They eventually took the pills off the market in the US (the European patent on the pill form was still in effect and no such "awareness campaign" took place there).
54. Christopher Moraff, "Suboxone Creator's Shocking Scheme to Profit Off of Heroin Addicts," *Daily Beast*, October 5, 2016, sec. US News, https://www.thedailybeast.com/articles/2016/10/05/suboxone-creator-said-its-pills-killed-kids-to-make-1-billion.

one same crisis conundrum in the quest for ever-growing profits on a finite planet. Rather than seeking an end to social ills and a cure for capitalism's produced articulations of harm, solutions from within the system's partitioned consciousness arise to contain and co-opt the self-perpetuating crises that threaten its survival, securing fixes that satiate, though never sufficiently, its constant quest for growth.

CHAPTER 8

BODIES IN REVOLT

The body is a precursor to consciousness.

—Cedric Robinson, *An Anthropology of Marxism* (2001)

From the dead but dominant paradigm's perspective, the whole world's a powder keg. Everything's about to blow. Chronic stress makes higher-order kinds of thought—such as curiosity, creativity, generosity, or grace—unavailable. The prefrontal cortex goes offline. The amygdala drives. We find ourselves scanning for, identifying, obsessing over, inventing, and reacting to threats. The breath constricts. The body tightens. We retreat from each other in fear, or band together in reactive mobs. The confluence of fright and threat makes us easy to manipulate with commodified info-tainment designed to keep us wanting one thing: more. This final chapter offers provocations and observations intended to encourage more interventions at the level of mass consciousness that produce new collective understandings of what needs changing. The same machinations that got the dislocated and disaffected masses hooked on pain pills now seeks to get them Red Pilled in the service of the system's bedrock asset: the capacity to wage all-out war in the service of endless accumulation. ·

REQUIEM FOR THE COGITO

I was 36 when I learned about the rest-and-digest nervous system state. I'd lived my whole life in fight-or-flight mode. The revelation came in the third hour of a three-hour back pain workshop at the Feldenkrais

Institute in New York City. Moshe Feldenkrais, a physicist and engineer and the developer of the Feldenkrais Method, identified socially engrained domination and suppression of individual spontaneity, particularly in the Western education system, as a pervasive cause of pain and pathology in the body. I left the workshop taking fuller, more natural breaths, and in considerably less pain than I'd been in in years. It was 2017, and in 2011 a Harvard-trained, Park Avenue rheumatologist recommended a patented, injectable immune suppressant drug for a condition that she said was progressive, degenerative, and irreversible. My immune system, she said, was eating my spine. "Without the medication, you will not walk by the time you're 40," she told me. I got a second opinion, which was, "You don't need this drug *yet. Save it for when you're worse.*" Neither doctor had any sense of how I might get *better.* This was my first clue that something might be wrong with their way of seeing me. Deep down, beneath all the pain and calcified fear, I could feel my capacity to regenerate and heal. I knew there was a strength and intelligence somewhere in this system, my living body, from which I'd spent most of my life estranged.

Silvia Federici writes of the project to dominate the human body and reproduce it in capital's image: "The body had to die so that labor power could live."[1] This partitioning of the living human organism into body and mind is of a piece with the broader project to erase our knowing and our capacities, in order that we might be dominated and controlled. Erasure, severing, and forced forgetting are necessary for turning the body, like the Earth, into terrain for endless war and extraction. The current Western medical system pursues problems in the body accordingly: pathologize, partition, contain.

Yet, the human body, like the Earth, defies carving up and compartmentalizing. Beginning in the mid-twentieth century, some Western theorists and healers started moving beyond the dead but dominant paradigm for the human body as an object among objects to an integrated somatic approach, which foregrounds the mind-body unity, and is focused on systems. For example, a somatic approach appreciates the nervous system as a sensory intelligence network that is inherently relational—both within the living organism and with the

---

1.   Silvia Federici, *Caliban and the Witch: Women, the Body, and Primitive Accumulation* (New York: Autonomedia, 2004).

outside world—and that unites what some refer to as the body's "three brains"—in the skull (and spinal column), the heart, and the gut.

In *Phenomenology of Perception* (1945), French philosopher Maurice Merleau-Ponty positions the body as an active participant in the perceptual process as opposed to being merely a passive receiver of sensations. Our bodily experiences and interactions with the world are presented as integral to how we think, perceive, and understand. The Cartesian view that prioritizes reason and cognition is challenged by Merleau-Ponty's understanding of how our bodily experiences shape our sensory understanding. He critiques Descartes' concept of the *cogito*, the idea that there is a level of awareness and experience that precedes thought and is deeply rooted in bodily experience, proposing instead the concept of a *pre-reflective consciousness*. Peter Levine, founder of Somatic Experiencing, a relationally based practice for resolving the remnants of embodied traumas, pushes this reframing of the cogito further: "I move, I sense, I feel, I perceive, and I reason, therefore I am alive and real."[2]

The grips of Cartesian mind-body duality, the naturalized violence within Western Enlightenment thought, the central conceits of liberal ideology—of who is and is not deserving of suffering—are all losing sway. Increasingly one's sensory perception of the world, one's lived experience as they are situated within this paradigm, calls on us to listen to the knowledge in our bodies, in our gut. We feel fueled and overwhelmed by this contrarian wisdom that rebels within us, that calls on us to ask the difficult questions, to reject simplistic historiographies that serve to naturalize and render invisible ongoing everyday acts of violence at a range of scales from the corporeal to the global.

It appears more humans than ever are finding it difficult to be here. The traumas we hold individually, and collectively, are immense. Some say anxiety is the "affect of the age" and an "open secret."[3] Others pinpoint hopelessness, depression, or "cruel optimism."[4] Capital thrives on the myth that we can satisfactorily escape human suffering

2. Peter Levine, "Trauma Stored in the Body: Somatic Experiencing," *Chasing Consciousness*, Episode 54, April 15, 2024, https://www.youtube.com/watch?v=GGLU9Xyu2DY.
3. Andrea Tone, *The Age of Anxiety: A History of America's Turbulent Affair with Tranquilizers* (New York: Basic Books 2012).
4. Lisa Duggan and José Esteban Muñoz, "Hope and Hopelessness: A Dialogue," *Women and Performance* 19, no. 2 (January 1, 2009): 275–283; Ann Cvetkovich, *Depression: A Public Feeling* (Durham: Duke University Press Books, 2012); Berlant, *Cruel Optimism*.

through participation in the market. Liberalism tells us that each of us is endowed with the capacity to turn our own fortunes using whatever resources are available to us, including other human beings; it provides the ideological contours for the socio-geographical distinction of waste and value, central to the valorization of capital.[5] This central affective conceit of capitalism not only ignores a basic tenet of life on Earth—some suffering is inevitable—it also externalizes the immense human suffering produced in capital's own image.

ALL THE RAGE: REBELLIOUS PAIN AND FASCISM

I imagine one of the reasons people cling to their hates so stubbornly is because they sense, once hate is gone, they will be forced to deal with their pain.

—James Baldwin

Hannah Arendt, Alice Miller, Wilhelm Reich, Eric Fromm, George Orwell, Theodor Adorno, Umberto Eco, and others explore the emotional, affective appeal of fascism and its corresponding psychological imprinting. At its core, the system's appeal rests in its emotionality. Fascist movements play into and seek resonance not with its form of "reason" as liberalism does, but with a collective's repressed and festering "negative" feeling states. Mind-body rage can express inward as pain or outward as violence.

Fascism taps the unpleasant emotions that are essential and unavoidable in a class society under capitalism. Shifting regimes of capital accumulation necessitate that the divided populace be reconfigured according to new circuits of production, circulation, and consumption. It necessitates that once-dominant groups be *denigrated*. While liberalism ignores and gaslights the fact that the system makes nearly everyone feel inadequate and vulnerable, even the ones it says are supposed to be "on top," fascism feeds on this fact. It speaks into the electrified forcefield of the voiceless, unnamed, atomized,

---

5.　Sharad Chari and Vinay Gidwani, "Introduction Grounds for a Spatial Ethnography of Labor," *Ethnography* 6, no. 3 (September 1, 2005): 267–281; Neil Smith, *The Endgame of Globalization* (New York: Routledge, 2003); Cindi Katz, "Vagabond Capitalism and the Necessity of Social Reproduction," in *Antipode* 33, no. 4 (2001): 709–728; James Ferguson, *The Anti-Politics Machine: Development, Depoliticization, and Bureaucratic Power in Lesotho* (Minneapolis: University of Minnesota Press, 1994).

alienated rebellion always under way. As ways of being and seeing get erased, the masses end up in an embodied state of emotional, social, and economic disempowerment. Fascism puts this unconscious disarticulated rebellion to work.

All humans seek to belong, to feel seen, to have their emotional state mirrored back to them in recognition. All humans want to know that no matter how bad they are feeling, they are good. German sociologist Arthur Rosenberg's 1934 article "Fascism as a Mass Movement" offers a crucial framing for understanding the rising popularity of fascist movements today.[6] In contrast to many theorists who argue that fascism is a top-down movement stirred by elements of the upper class seeking to compel the masses to their cause of reorganizing capital to suit their class consolidation, Rosenberg posits—as the title suggests—that the real story for understanding the appeal of the ideology stems organically from the populace.

These feeling states do not need to be manufactured. Fascism spreads like wildfire, he says, because it speaks to an unspoken core in dislocated, disturbed, dispossessed people who had, in a previous era of economic accumulation, been told they were on top, were the nation's pride and joy, were the heart of the machine. Elements of the upper class seize the opportunity presented by the presence of—and mainstream liberal disavowal of—these sentiments. In other words, class power manipulates but does not manufacture the discontent. The sentiments are real, organically existing among the masses and seeking, as all energy does, an outlet, a course, a direction. The real cause of mass repressed rage, in the hermeneutic vacuum of the dead but dominant paradigm, goes undiagnosed. This leaves the masses certain that a fix is in, distrustful of the system and one another, frightened and thus operating from lower-order cognition; not the higher consciousness that can see parts of a whole, but the amygdala, whose fight, flight, freeze, or fawn response can be and is coopted by capital.

Alice Miller and Wilhelm Reich posit that the affective allure of fascism originates in deep hurts; often in childhood wounding. In severing our very selves into incommensurable parts, the system puts the fact of our integral mind-body unity to work against us. Hermeneutic

---

6.   Arthur Rosenberg, "Fascism as a Mass-Movement (1934)," *Historical Materialism* 20, no. 1 (January 1, 2012): 144–189.

violence is erasure, the production of black holes in the collective's capacity to see what's going on while the system slurps more of our lifeforce, through trickery, obfuscation, and other parlor tricks of partitioned consciousness. Through our partitioned collective consciousness, the harm embedded in the system is splintered off in our causal understandings. The externalized violence of the system becomes internalized in our bodies, minds, and spirits.

Arthur Sackler absolutely understood the mind-body unity. Social media firms (private-sector and state-backed technologies alike) also exploit this knowingness. Technological advances in the profit- and power-centric paradigm innovate ways to capture our consciousness. Deep fake videos, combined with algorithmic means to not only cater to a user's affective disposition but to change it, are intensifying the rising trend of mis- and disinformation contributing to the erosion of meaning and fractured claims to reality.

New York Times podcast series *Rabbit Hole* offers a compelling exploration of the Internet's power to shape our lives, beliefs, and society, often in ways we're not fully aware. It illustrates how algorithms, particularly those used by platforms like YouTube, can influence users' thinking and behavior. It shows how these algorithms, built as weapons in the war for attention, which in the digital advertising landscape where the data gathered on our behavior online is the commodity for sale, by design introduce users of the drug, I mean technology, to increasingly extreme or polarizing content. These algorithms are attributable to the severe and significant radicalization and consciousness programming that became evident in the COVID-19 pandemic. One illustration of this is the phenomena dubbed Pastel Q, named after the Q Anon conspiracy, one of the major motivating factors behind the January 6, 2021 Capitol Riots. Pastel Q refers to the thousands of American women in their thirties consuming health, fitness, and holistic mothering content who were funneled into anti-vax-Rothschilds-adrenochrome kinds of content, swallowing the proverbial Red Pill.

Importantly, this experience is another instance of being stuck in capital's fix, reproduced as *tierra firma*, that which can be extracted from. It amounts to a person's life force having been hijacked. This, like the profit-driven logic of the morphine molecule, makes our embodied consciousness a fix for capital and the state (and, more significantly, vying global factions seeking to destroy or become a given state formation, 'winning hearts and minds' by any means necessary). Just like supply-side hooks might find a person starting with a prescription from the doctor for oxycodone only months later copping street-supplied fentanyl, millions of people found themselves researching garlic as a home remedy for immune support and learning instead a wild tale putting George Soros at the top of some bloodsucking cabal or another. Addressing social media's addictive intention in a July 2023 *Washington Post* interview, Anna Lembke, Medical Director of Addictive Medicine at Stanford, said that the industry "has essentially taken human connection and turned it into a drug by distilling it down to the essential properties that make something addictive."[7] In *The Chaos Machine*, Max Fisher quotes an internal Facebook memo that put the matter succinctly: "Our algorithms exploit the human brain's attraction to divisiveness."[8]

NOSTALGIA, DISLOCATION, AND TRAPPED RAGE

Chinese peasant mythology includes a tale about the origins of opium:

The story tells of a man with a very ugly wife who upset him so that he could do nothing but curse her and threaten to throw her out. The wife accepted his ill-treatment, for she loved him dearly; but finally, she fell ill of despair. As the hour of her death approached she said to her husband that despite the evil way in which he had treated her, he would realize after her death how much she loved him. About a week after her burial the husband learnt that a beautiful white flower had appeared on her grave. Within the flower was a small round fruit. This curious phenomenon worried the widower, who remembered the dying woman's words and began to regret his ill-behavior. He wondered whether she had turned into a plant in order to injure him. Finally, thoughts of his dead wife so filled his mind that he could neither sleep nor work. He fell ill, but he had no children to care for him, nor could the doctors help him. Then one night his wife appeared to him in a dream. She told him that the plant

---

7. Luis Velarde, "How Addictive, Endless Scrolling Is Bad for Your Mental Health," *Washington Post*, July 14, 2023, https://www.washingtonpost.com/science/2023/07/14/social-media-mental-crisis-youths/.

8. Max Fisher, *The Chaos Machine: The Inside Story of How Social Media Rewired Our Minds and Our World* (New York: Little, Brown and Company, 2022).

on her grave was formed from her soul: from a cut in the central fruit a
juice would appear which, once it had hardened, could be smoked in a
pipe. If her husband smoked the juice every day he would be relieved of
his suffering.[9]

Central to the condition of addiction is the desire to return to an irreconcilable past, to recover that which has been lost and cannot be regained. From Canton to Weimar to Vietnam to Harlem and Harlan County, opioids/opiates earn their keep by quelling inconsolable pain, making despair more tolerable, and providing a modicum of comfort in palliative care. The conceit in Purdue's ad campaign, that opioids promise a better future, goes against the biomolecular fact of the drug itself, which blunts one's capacity to have any regard for the future.

Yet, in its debut campaign in 1996, Purdue marketed OxyContin as if it was about returning to life before pain. One early ad showed an older man on the golf course, with the tagline: "Get back into the swing of things with OxyContin!"[10] Promotional material included a CD of danceable tunes and a sun visor. The image the company constructed was about the *life-giving* promise of the drug, which would encourage ease of movement and a return to work and play. As the ink was drying on deepening rounds of the NAFTA deal, and as American jobs were lost to technological innovation or else shipped to places with far lower wage rates and no such thing as costly unions, worker's rights or labor standards, most Americans in pain found themselves stuck in place without a life to get back to.

In their measured assessment of the factors contributing to the opioid epidemic, public health scholars Nabarun Dasgupta, Leo Beletsky, and Daniel Ciccarone challenge the dominant "bad apple" (Sackler) and "demon-drug" (Oxy) narratives. "Although drug supply is a key factor, we posit that the crisis is fundamentally fueled by economic and social upheaval, its etiology closely linked to the role of opioids as a refuge from physical and psychological trauma, concentrated disadvantage, isolation, and hopelessness."[11] The lived experience

---

9.   Anthony Christine, *Chinese Peasant Mythology* (London: Hamlyn Publishing Group, 1968).
10.   Van Zee, "The Promotion and Marketing of OxyContin."
11.   Nabarun Dasgupta, Leo Beletsky, and Daniel Ciccarone, "Opioid Crisis: No Easy Fix to Its Social and Economic Determinants," *American Journal of Public Health* 108, no. 2 (February

of the financial squeeze and economic dislocation of the American working class produced a silent epidemic of suffering. Without political consensus or salient frameworks for a coherent shared critique, the shame-based, isolating disciplinary logic of *Homo economicus* produced an epidemic of private, individuated pain and suffering for the multiracial American working class.

From within this variegated landscape of embodiment and lived experience, those with a predilection to consider that what had been before was better than the present turned what otherwise could have been fodder for a collective revolutionary imaginary instead into a wistful longing to return to the past. In her 1999 memoir *How to Stop Time*, Ann Marlowe writes, "If I had to offer up a one sentence definition of addiction, I'd call it a form of mourning for the irrecoverable glories of the first time. This means that addiction is essentially nostalgic, which ought to tarnish the luster of nostalgia as much as that of addiction. Addiction can show us what is deeply suspect about nostalgia. That drive to return to the past isn't an innocent one. It's about stopping your passage to the future, it's a symptom of fear of death, and the love of predictable experiences."[12]

The origins of the word nostalgia speak to this. It was invented to define a medical condition, a cluster of symptoms observed in the seventeenth century by a Swiss medical student named Johannes Hofer. Hofer observed physical and sometimes fatal symptoms in his patients that stemmed from a form of extreme homesickness. In 1688, he named the condition "nostalgia," combining the Greek words *nostos* [homecoming] and *alga* [pain].[13]

People who succumb to opioid dependence display a longing to return to a past that cannot be retrieved, whether because things were better there, or because an injustice occurred there that lingers in one's present, that keeps one from attending to the present, that one returns to in their mind in the hopes of making it right, of seeing how it could have gone differently. Whether personal or structural, this type of injury to the soul, a reality that went against the promise,

2018): 182–186.
12. Marlowe, *How to Stop Time*, 10.
13. Adrienne Matei, "Nostalgia's Unexpected Etymology Explains Why It Can Feel so Painful," *Quartz*, October 22, 2017, https://qz.com/1108120/nostalgias-unexpected-etymology-explains-why-it-can-feel-so-painful/.

expectations, of life, seems to animate habituation to and deleterious use of pain-numbing drugs. In a study on "complicated grief," medical doctor and neurobiologist M. Katherine Shear explains the bio-emotional feedback spiral that can turn feelings of loss into rage and other painful feeling states: "Complicating emotional processes are negative valence emotions such as guilt, envy, bitterness, or anger, that are relentlessly activated and excessively painful, without periods of respite from positive emotions."[14]

Nostalgia and wishing to return to an idealized past, amidst a present that is unmanageable and a future that is unimaginable[15]—these affective traits are pervasive in the present. Nostalgia is correlated with scarcity consciousness and a lack of trust in the present. It is for this affective-material-embodied set of reasons that nostalgia is a central feature of both opioid use disorder and totalitarian, populist, right-wing ideology. Nostalgia is a key characteristic of the consciousness, sense of life, and the world of those who are willing to subscribe to a reactionary ideology. Mark Lila's 2016 *The Shipwrecked Mind* and Corey Robin's 2011 *The Reactionary Mind* both focus centrally on the toxic manifestations of nostalgia, a predisposition to focus on a past where things were better or could have gone differently.[16] These emotional traits are central to the covert and well-funded campaigns to get the masses drafted onto one side or another, it doesn't matter which one, rooting for war.

The intensification of rates of extraction often coincide historically with the extension of formal rights and gestures of 'progressive' inclusion.[17] David Graeber demonstrates that debt is a tool of imperial domination that can exist among people who are formally equals.[18] Debt and addiction proliferation amidst the kind of inequality that can

---

14. M. Katherine Shear, "Grief and Mourning Gone Awry: Pathway and Course of Complicated Grief," *Dialogues in Clinical Neuroscience* 14, no. 2 (June 1, 2012): 119–128.

15. Paraphrasing Jennifer DiSilva, *Coming Up Short: Working-Class Adulthood in an Age of Uncertainty* (Oxford: Oxford University Press, 2014).

16. Corey Robin, *The Reactionary Mind: Conservatism from Edmund Burke to Sarah Palin* (Oxford: Oxford University Press, 2013); Mark Lilla, *The Shipwrecked Mind: On Political Reaction* (New York: New York Review Books, 2016).

17. Melamed, "The Spirit of Neoliberalism from Racial Liberalism to Neoliberal Multiculturalism"; Melamed, *Represent and Destroy*; Nikhil Pal Singh, *Black Is a Country: Race and the Unfinished Struggle for Democracy* (Cambridge: Harvard University Press, 2005).

18. Graeber, *Debt*; Annie Spencer, "Woman Is an Object Without History (and Other Reflections upon Reading David Graeber's Debt: The First 5,000 Years)," *Women's Studies Quarterly* 42, no. 1/2 (April 1, 2014): 38–45.

masquerade as justice, can be outsourced and displaced onto individuals who can be blamed. Debt relations, addiction, and moralism proliferate and individuate amidst the intensification of neoliberalism's extractivist foreclosure of ways of life.

PATHOLOGIZE, PARTITION, CONTAIN

"*Cogito, ergo sum*" ["I think, therefore I am"] appears first in Descartes' "Discourse on the Method" (1637) and more formally in "Meditations on First Philosophy" (1641). The premise suggests intelligence rests in "the mind" and the body is a bit like a machine driven by the human, who is, in the common-sense perspective of the dead but dominant paradigm, the mind.

In the dominant tradition of Western thought the beingness of a person is identified with the mind and the body is either absent or treated as unintelligent. This knowledge system, a product of the European Enlightenment, privileges facts and figures over instincts, perceptions, ancestral wisdom, and body knowledge—gut feelings and other information inferred by the nervous system, which is a relational intelligence system. Erasing our collective memory and ways of knowing of a life outside the profit motive's twisted logic is central to the project of instantiating market, money, and profit-based social relation. In the absence of recognition of these other ways of knowing, the paradigm can reduce the fact of our unequal exchange to an equation, disappearing our capacity to evidence that which was taken unjustly. Biomedicine, psychiatry, economics, industrialism, monocropping, and other conventions of the dead but dominant world disorder split the mind from the body and the soul. In the project to split human beings from each other and the Earth, warfare is the method. At every scale, it imbues the dead but dominant paradigm.

In *When The Body Says No*, Gabor Maté discusses a host of mind-body illnesses and says that mind-body medicine remains a "Bermuda Triangle" in medical research.[19] In the absence of a unified conception of the living human organism, the system diagnoses what it sees as discrete failure with no clear cause or resolution. Chronic conditions

---

19. Gabor Maté, *When the Body Says No: The Cost of Hidden Stress* (Vancouver: Wiley, 2003).

are conceptualized as such because the medical system divides us into parts the same way the economic system divides us against each other. Sick people make a for-profit medical system more money than healthy ones. Chronic conditions are another way the system maintains, keeping us locked in its vice, conscripted to a painful reality, where all we can hope for is commodified relief.

TRAPPED RAGE EXPRESSED

We forget how long abuses can continue 'unknown' until they are articulated: how people can look at misery and not notice it, until misery itself rebels.

—E.P. Thompson, *The Making of the English Working Class* (1963)

In the same year as my diagnosis, the US Institute of Medicine (IOM) report "Relieving Pain in America: A Blueprint for Transforming Prevention, Care, Education, and Research" identified an epidemic of chronic pain affecting nearly a third of all Americans.[20] The startling conclusions of the IOM pain report prompted a 2012 hearing, "Pain in America," convened by the Senate Committee on Health, Education, Labor, and Pensions. During the hearing, a particularly powerful exchange occurred between Senator Bernie Sanders and Dr. John E. Sarno, Professor of Rehabilitation Medicine at New York University School of Medicine and attending physician at the Howard A. Rusk Institute of Rehabilitation Medicine.

Dr. Sarno, who passed in 2017 at the age of ninety-four, was an innovative researcher, practitioner, and author whose unorthodox theory and methods have helped thousands of patients find resolution from pain for which medical orthodoxy offered no solution.[21] Sarno's approach uncovered the hidden psychological roots to chronic and often severe physical pain. In what he named Tension Myositis Syndrome (TNS), Sarno posited that the epidemic of chronic physical pain

---

20. Institute of Medicine (US) Committee on Advancing Pain Research, "Relieving Pain in America: A Blueprint for Transforming Prevention, Care, Education, and Research," 2011, https://www.ncbi.nlm.nih.gov/books/NBK92510/.
21. John E. Sarno, *Healing Back Pain: The Mind-Body Connection* (New York: Warner Books, 1991); John E. Sarno, *The Mindbody Prescription: Healing the Body, Healing the Pain* (New York: Warner Books, Inc., 1999); John E. Sarno, *The Divided Mind: The Epidemic of Mindbody Disorders* (New York: Harper Perennial, 2007).

results from suppressed psychological tension—stress, rage, fear, and other painful emotions. Finding commonality with a host of other psychosomatic conditions, Sarno theorized that chronic physical pain results from the unconscious mind's accessing of the autonomic nervous system. He saw this as a coping mechanism for emotional pain that the conscious mind is unwilling or unable to express.[22] Sarno said that his understanding of the unconscious mind's manifestation of physical ailments relating to suppressed emotions were connected to an observation about the virtual disappearance of ulcers, once a ubiquitous health complaint, as soon as it was raised to popular consciousness that ulcers were stress-related.[23]

Sarno theorized that chronic pain, in the form of chronic muscle and fascia tension resulting from autonomic nervous system activation from stress, became the new, predominant pathway for suppressed stress and rage to manifest in the body. Another expert testifying in the 2012 Senate hearing, Duke University Professor of Anesthesiology and Co-Director for the Center for Translational Pain Medicine, William Maixner, stated that, "socioeconomic status may even be a surrogate marker of environmental exposures" and susceptibility to chronic pain. Elucidating the mind-body unity and speaking on the phenomena of somatized social pain sweeping the country, Sarno said, "Poor people are angry, furious as a matter of fact at what society has allowed to happen. That fury will provoke symptomatology, believe it or not, that is a defense against the rage. They can't rage, and so, what happens is that they get sick, and I believe that this is an extremely common phenomenon." Senator Sanders replied, "You mean, rather than burning down the Capitol, they are turning that anger against themselves, right?" To which Dr. Sarno replies, "Exactly."

I recall Chris Hedges' unheeded warning to a packed auditorium at the Graduate Center in 2011 about the need for a movement that spoke to the masses: someone is going to coopt the mass discontent of this country.

---

22. Sarno, *The Mindbody Prescription*; John W. Burns, "Arousal of Negative Emotions and Symptom-Specific Reactivity in Chronic Low Back Pain Patients," *Emotion (Washington, D.C.)* 6, no. 2 (May 2006): 309–319.
23. Russell Baker, "Where Have All the Ulcers Gone?," *New York Times*, August 16, 1981, sec. Magazine, https://www.nytimes.com/1981/08/16/magazine/sunday-observer-where-have-all-the-ulcers-gone.html; Sarno, *The Mindbody Prescription*.

Who will it be next?

CONCLUSION

The essence of revolution is not the struggle for bread; it is the struggle for human dignity.

—Adolfo Gilly, introduction to Franz Fanon's
A Dying Colonialism (1959)

ROCK BOTTOM

Behind the curtain of the dead and dying world disorder is a math equation pretending it can 'make up' for what's been taken. A "my bad, we'll tweak the formula" is the dead but dominant system's reply to being called out for having turned our Mother into Money. All the world's hungry horde of capital lurches now in a mad dash for a chunk of the real base, a pound of flesh or a parcel of Earth. *La tierra firma.* In the final act, it is our Earth mother, and her life-forms, that have what the system needs. *Value.*

It's dog eat dog out there, and Big Dog, General Dynamics' robotic pack animal, is patrolling the southern US border. The Chinese military, I read this morning, is conducting exercises with the Belarusian army on the Polish border. The horror in Gaza wages on. We've breached 1.5 C. Somehow, we're supposedly electing a new American president this November. The number of migrants worldwide seeking safe haven is intensifying as is dehumanizing rhetoric and violence against them. Everybody knows it's Go Time, but *go where* time?

Capitalism requires compounding immiseration, period. In its defense of the system, liberalism holds the door for fascism. Totalitarian state capitalist regimes waving red stars and the banner of Karl Marx are no different from Christian fascists acting like they've got something to do with the teachings of Christ. And the liberals, with their false god of morality and 'reason,' have the best disguise of all. Transcending dualism means learning to see that fascism and liberalism are two sides of the same shit-eating coin of imperialism's long march to planetary ruin. Liberalism depends on fascism. It has never been a viable challenge to it. Together liberalism and fascism create the cat and mouse game, the revolving door of imperialist formations of disordered order, contorted logic, and misplaced meaning that keep us all on its hook, fighting its, instead of our own, fight.

Writing this book has had so much to do with my inner life, with my pain, my trapped rage. I don't only mean around my mother and brother getting hooked on opioids, but other things too. Like my early childhood experience being the one in charge of stopping outbreaks of domestic war. When you're a child, your family is your world, and so the weight of world war grew on my chest, my spine, my mind, as my consciousness expanded and I saw further and more grotesque articulations of the same tendencies at larger scales. My mother's demons preferred to start a war rather than be found out. Warfare was a diversionary tactic meant to throw everyone, including her, off the trail of what grew stronger in the shadow of her unconscious, *that which could not be named*. The secrets she lived her life unable to unburden herself of, the shame she could never slay, the rage she struggled to find the right outlet for, became the bedrock of our existence. And then I became a strange loop.

What we resist persists, the "Twelve Step" adage goes. What we ignore, hoping to avoid the consequences of needing to face—even if we didn't create it—grows stronger, as if self-aware of the power it has over us in our fear of it.

Is your nervous system activated by all the rumble and all the rubble? Thinking about some commodified relief? Got some psychic tension you'd like to reduce? Let's recite the Serenity Prayer together:

God,[1] grant me the serenity to accept the things I cannot change, the courage to change the things I can, and the wisdom to know the difference.

THE WISDOM TO KNOW THE DIFFERENCE

David Harvey is in my ear: "*In the final act, who is holding the gun?*" How do we catch the tiger by the tail, see capital in motion as it shifts shape, makes its moves for another Grand Golpe? *Who done it?* Who is doing it, and what will it take to break the addiction, this world-scale dependency that deteriorates?

Knowing the difference means knowing where we stand. Reading the landscape, we are equipped with a map sufficiently detailed to help us recognize, evoking Prince, the patron saint of this work, the signs of the times. I pulled on the opioid epidemic and unraveled present-day imperialism sufficiently enough to understand where I stand. What problem keeps you up at night? What wants a piece of you, a pound of your flesh? What issue bites into your existence, to paraphrase Ruth Wilson Gilmore? We've reached a point where the convergence of crises exposes our commonalities. The fact is, our struggles are bound up in one another's, and the only thing we have to lose—evoking Marx, Engels and Assata Shakur, is our chains. The question then becomes, how do we change everything?

The species-defining challenge of the present moment will not be solved by political ideology or technological development, but through the emergence of a new collective consciousness. The crack in the wall, to evoke the 2015 communique from Subcomandante Galeano,[2] is a portal to another spacetime reality, where more dimensions of understanding, more context to what is known and believed to be relevant and true, exists. Cedric Robinson taught in *Black Marxism* that the creation of new theory requires new histories. Geographer Clyde Woods taught me to understand theory-making as indistinct from

---

1. This word can be replaced with Higher Power, the Great Mystery, Ancestors, Gaia, Divine Intelligence, Higher Self—whatever reminds you that the voice talking in your head is NOT the sum of who you are nor is it the most intelligent force in the universe. How's that for a rational thought?
2. Subcomandante Insurgente Galeano, "The Crack in the Wall. First Note on Zapatista Method," Mexico, May 3, 2015, https://enlacezapatista.ezln.org.mx/2015/05/10/the-crack-in-the-wall-first-note-on-zapatista-method/.

storytelling. Dancing the dialectic of new histories and new theories allows us to weave tapestries in new dimensions. Weaving new space-time grids, we chart new and revolutionary courses. Our new maps make available new territory, new topography—reaching, evoking Stevie Wonder, higher ground.

The tricky thing about present-day imperialism is that just as often and as significant as all the external forces exerting domination and keeping us captive, is the wizard behind the curtain in our own heads. Our partitioned minds keep us unfree. It's apparently a self-protective mechanism. The mind hides the truth from us because it thinks, in doing so, that it is keeping us safe. But safety, like abstract value, is an illusion. The truth is something more complex that exists only between us.

The present articulations of premeditated and preventable harm, the rampant expulsion of life, health, harmony, and thriving share a common cause that can be seen only in the light of a new *way of seeing*, a new paradigm. This is at once a geographical project and a question of perception. The truth is true because we can locate, in its context, ourselves and all the rest of who and what exists. The inverse is the dialectic that tests the premise: in order to know what is true, we must know who and where we are. We must locate ourselves at a world-scale in a quantum field, as a constant and constantly changing part to the whole of what exists—in space, time, and matter.

New ways of seeing render visible not only new histories and understandings about how the present came to pass but makes possible, legible, attainable new theories and imaginaries for world-making, beyond the present conjuncture of crises. Consciousness expansion is the work of building bridges in our knowledge and understanding. From new vantages we see more clearly the lay of the land and gain necessary perspective from which to formulate an adequately different vision for human collective life lived otherwise.

LOOPS VS. SPIRALS

That which is not conscious operates on a pattern, through default programing and perpetual motion. Its story is already written. It has a destiny. Consciousness produces awareness; it creates a field of possibility into which the conscious actor might inject a choice. This is agency; the application of presence, intention, and energy applied at a given location in a given direction. These are spatial considerations. Capitalism is not a conspiracy. It is an operating system. Like any other, it can be uninstalled. Everything can change. All our intelligence and networks and ways of being together can be replaced with something better, something new.

What is needed now is not a midpoint or a compromise, but a quantum leap in our collective consciousness and thus our capacity, our species potential. A new vector, a location, another third thing. The difference is scalar and dimensional. In its many dimensions, it is also relational. It is not static; it is in motion, like a river. The space-time of revolution is a plane of possibility. The journey to get there is a dialectical inquiry that unfolds from that which calls you from your soul in the night.

There is no Grand Conspiracy. There is instead series of strange loops we're stuck in because we can't remember how we got here, what came before, what and how else we otherwise might be. There is good and evil, loving and hateful intent, but what there mostly are are games people play. How do we change the game? How do we take power? How do we imagine power beyond this ugly game's version of it, as something holy and in common, like the power of the Earth herself? How do we decompose capital and arrive back at a living Earth, part of it, parts to our own and each other's sentient whole? I don't know the answers, but having settled into a spontaneous deep sigh while asking, I know my soma likes this line of questioning.

BODY KNOWING

The colonial knowledge paradigm has left us estranged from, if not enemies to, our living soma. We've forgotten the body's language, that it has wisdom. It all goes back to the pound of flesh, the parcel of land, that which can be carved up, owned, held because it is said to have value. Getting uncolonized means in part undoing thousands of years of epigenetic imprinting in the service of our domination, the breaking of our spirit. It means coming home to our living, breathing, intelligent organisms, the soma, the sensing, perceiving, re-membering

being. You've gotta be in your body in order to come home. It's collective work. It can't be done alone.

I lived in fight-or-flight most of my life. And I came from my
mother's body, and it was that way there too. Humans make decisions based on instincts, information and perception, but when fear
is in the mix, the calculations can be ungrounded. The energy of fear
detaches us from a felt sense of our connection to our surroundings.
Destabilization is a key tactic of colonization. It is is the necessary
act that enables so-called primitive accumulation, *golpe growth.* The
Earth quakes beneath our feet, while our will is hijacked by our neurochemistry to a conveniently unimaginative and pliable choice set, right
where capital's agents want us: *fight, flight, freeze, or fawn.*

HOW TO JUMP SCALE

*Thus objective social realities of the time overtook the conventional wisdom and
served to expose its failings.*

—David Harvey, "Revolutionary and Counter Revolutionary
Theory in Geography" (1972)

My health conditions, which I'm still learning to manage, turned out
to be about the relational systems of the soma, in particular the nervous system and the fascia. It is only looking back on the completed
text that I see I made a book that works a bit like connective tissue
too. My obsession this lifetime: amidst all that would seek to break
us apart, what is it that holds us together? How do we see it enough
to value it enough to choose it? After all this short-run conditioning,
fear-based programming, and disciplining of our imaginative capacity,
curiosity, and sight, what is it going to take to get us to choose to try for
something better (speculative, make-believe) instead?

Have you heard the moon is getting a time zone? There's so much
commercial traffic up there these days, did you notice? Not just for
fun, but for the same reasons European ships set sail back in 1492.
Private firms, bankrolled by billionaires, are casing the joint, planning
mining operations. The flurry of traffic and plans for extractive operations is being called an "interstellar armada." The seabed floor too is
being mined. What was once considered a flat surface is being opened

up to further dimensions. The old world's idea of quantum isn't just an innovation in computational speed. New dimensions of reality are being introduced. But alas, until we change it, these frontiers are being shaped in capital's image. *Better, cheaper, faster. Short-term, high-yield. No pain, no gain. Pump it, dump it, strip it, seize it. Here today; gone tomorrow.*

My brother Michael, who died in 2005, was a huge Star Trek fan. He used to predict that peace on Earth would come about when we learned of extraterrestrial life, some sudden introduction of an off planet intelligent life force would allow for a unified identity among the human race, he'd say, while we watched the terrible news of the terrible Bush years, back when we thought that was as bad as things could get. It's a scalar theory of identity, class, and solidarity. When the terrain shifts, our sense of ourselves too, must jump scale. He died the week his two-years-in-waiting disability application was approved. The first thing he bought with his check, besides Philadelphia Eagles shirts for the whole family, was a nice telescope.

We're still waiting on this kind of alien contact, but present-day world war and climate collapse do bring their own stark relief of a set of planetary pickles we must get to solving, in common. The invocation is not at all intended to erase all the significant social topographies, structural inequalities, among us Earthlings, but does bring into sharp contrast who and what we have in common, what time it is, what the stakes are.

CONSCIOUSNESS AND REVOLUTION

Consciousness is a social relation. It can spread like any other epidemic.[3] Revolutions in thought occur when the sum total of that which cannot be explained or adequately addressed by the dominant thought paradigm accumulates to the point that it can no longer be brushed off as an outlier or anomaly. What does it take to build a movement for everyone? How do we build a movement on the basis of what we have in common while being accountable to all that is and has been

3. Peter Haggett, *The Geographical Structure of Epidemics* (Oxford: Oxford University Press, 2000).

different? The degrees of privilege and personhood, group-differentiated subjugation to favor, punishment, and extermination granted under the colonial disorder? How do we build a movement that affirms the right to dignity for everyone, and is inoculated against the myriad tricks aimed to get us to divide and fight amongst ourselves over the scraps? How do we make space for, honor, and alchemize our rage? How do we use rage as a fuel for revolution rather than letting it get coopted to fuel capital's quest for more profit and plunder?

Amidst the collective experience of foreclosure and impasse, I've been given a puzzle of my own. My consciousness, my body, my being *don't work* in this old, sick world. I've been tasked with creating spaces, new games, new means by which to make life. My body, my life's greatest teacher, has me thinking about connective tissue, flexible infrastructure, integration. I've been playing with new shapes, new formations amidst the present's shifting temporalities and scales, the quaking spacetime of revolution. An intention to teach the paradigm shift, contribute this way of seeing to the ongoing and busy work of building truly mass movements, has me curious about perspectives and offerings that speak to the masses, that create a container from which we can hold the whole thing, or at least enough, in motion, to gesture at wholeness. I've been thinking about Maya Angelou's instructions to us in her inauguration poem, "On the Pulse of Morning," which was the only good thing the Clintons ever gave us: "*Give birth again to the dream. . . . Sculpt it into the image of your most public self.*"

In the perhaps too-grand gesture of calling this work a manifesto, I'm poking and provoking at something like a reinvigorated global class consciousness. Off the Blue Team/Red Team spectrum to say the least, it's *another, third thing*, a third place. You get there through that crack in the wall. I'm imagining everyone I might reach, who might see their very different story in the one I've put together here. I'm thinking of an ancestor of our movement who made the inverse transatlantic migratory path as me, Swedish American, troubadour-organizer, Joe Hill. I'm day-dreaming of something like One Big Union, an identity formation in the making, as we make together new kinds of collective being and action.

Me and all my friends on five continents and counting don't want any more war. We'd rather have a party instead. I'm starting a project called The We Know How to Party. It's a global political party for pro-Earth Earthlings. It's an organization for Earthlings returning home to ourselves, to our integrated soma and social bodies, to being a part of the ecosystem, after a very long exile. I've started a second book about it, *The We Know How To Party Program*. It's a book of policy for Earthlings, some notions on becoming ecosystemic, thoughts on how we might compost capital to arrive back home to ourselves and our living Earth Mother.

The We Know How to Party is a popular education project and a production company. It is a place to come together to learn and to unlearn the damaging discipline of the schooling regime. It is a flexible body with brand recognition that disarms the old presumptions of binary, warfare, algorithmic consciousness in the service of making more space for cognition, for recognition, for connection. It's a humble little upstart with global ambitions. It's my art project. It's a mystery school. Evoking the great wisdom of the great Dubois, *call it whatever, just get it done.* As for its organizational structure, for now it's my thing. I'm the Steve Jobs. But maybe someday we'll collectivize it. Is it real? Having put together the case in the preceding pages, I offer an impudent smirk in reply. It's as real as Econ 101.

RECOVERY AND REVOLUTIONARY SPACETIME

In all my many moves since I started my PhD program in 2010, I've kept a hold of a photocopied diagram David Harvey passed out in either his *Grundrisse* or *Capital Volume II* course. It is a spacetime grid with nine boxes, three vertical and three horizontal rows, reproduced from his book *Spaces of Global Capitalism*.[4] I've understood it to be a significant key to what I was learning to see, to theorize, to enact into being. It's always been at hand, on or near my desk. At some point, probably back in my Maine days, I scrawled on it in red pen, "*THIS IS A MAP*," and at another point I've circled the bottom, right square, which is the vector corresponding to "Relational Space (Time)" and "Spaces of Representation (lived space)." The box reads "visions, fantasies,

---

4. David Harvey, *Spaces of Global Capitalism: Towards a Theory of Uneven Geographical Development* (London and New York: Verso, 2006), 143.

desires, frustrations, memories, dreams, phantasms, psychic states."
Next to it, I've written in hot pink pen, "*Revolutionary Imaginaries.*"

Learning to see in greater depth and dimension has allowed me
to theorize into this spacetime, for myself and the collective. I think of
the process in the way Audre Lorde taught us to appreciate poetry, as a
first attempt at finding language for something that hasn't quite been
fully formed as a concept yet. The finding of the words (the shape, the
space, the sound, the container) is a bit like spinning cotton candy
from sugar-water vapor. Bit by bit, something materializes, takes form
that can be recognized, as if from nothing. This is the creative act.
This is the rabbit-in-a-hat magic trick of revolution. Revolutions happen in increments and leaps and bounds. As Lenin said, there are
decades where nothing happens, and days where decades happen. If
it seems a bit mystical, it is. Revolution is the work of applied faith:
attention, intention, action.

Recovery is the revolutionary leap in the collective consciousness
where we remember our belonging to an integral whole, where we
practice being together again, where we have faith in our collective
capacity to create, to pull off something beautiful, to win. Learning
new ways of seeing renders visible not only new histories and understandings about the present but new theories for imagining and
world-making, conceiving of a future beyond the present cluster of
crises, the myriad articulated instances of impasse to life and thriving.
The project of developing new capacity for (in)sight, the expansion of
our collective consciousness, is the work of building bridges from our
knowledge and questioning about the present here-and-now to other
dimensions in space and time. It is the work of training our sight for
pattern recognition as well as engaging with legacies of thought that
allow us to stitch new patterns into new constellations, new infrastructures for new expressions and collective meaning-making.

Colonization is any kind of unfreedom that becomes systemic,
engrained, and contains within it a power structure that is maintained
by a misperception, a pageantry, a false belief, an erasure, something
dynamic that has been made flat. Liberation is the dance of waking
each other from this deathly stupor. Beneath its moralism and divisiveness, behind ranking us as more or lesser, deserving or undeserving, beyond its retorts to a reductive, economistic, tit-for-tat rationale,
under its appeals to our base survival instincts and manipulation of

our sentiments and neurobiology, all this way of being has to defend itself is violence. It wants us to think this is all we are, all life has to offer—that at our core, this is our 'nature.' But we know better than this. Maybe drugs helped us learn. Or maybe it was a flower, a bird, a kind mentor, a child, our inner quiet knowing, or an ecstatic non-drug experience. But we know something else, something beautiful—possibility, solidarity, belonging, collaborative ingenuity—is within our collective power to summon into being. There's infinite possible worlds beyond this one. Infinite quantum games to play. When and where we unite, we have the power.

Let's end this Endless World War Machine. Let's get free.

About the Author

Annie Xibos Spencer was born in North Philadelphia and grew up in Venice, Florida. They studied economics and international studies at New College of Florida and Latin American political economy at La Universidad de Belgrano in Buenos Aires. Their undergraduate honors thesis on the role of the IMF in the Argentine Peso Crisis earned them a job at the World Bank Institute where they worked as a writer and program evaluator while obtaining a MA in International Trade and Investment Policy at George Washington University. Spencer spent two summers in Dhaka, Bangladesh on a fellowship where she studied Bengali language and culture at the Independent University of Bangladesh and learned from feminist-Marxist agrarian movement, Naya Krishi Andolon. Spencer was an active participant in Occupy Wall Street and a founding member of the Occupy Student Debt Campaign and STRIKE Debt.

Spencer has worked in mutual-aid harm reduction and organized on the opioid epidemic and against state abandonment of people who use drugs in Maine. In 2020 they completed a PhD in human geography from the City University of New York (CUNY) Graduate Center, where they won the 2017 Provost's Award for Scholarship in the Public Interest and the 2016 Revolutionizing American Studies dissertation award. Spencer was a doctoral fellow with the Center for Place, Culture and Politics and the Mellon Committee on Globalization and Social Change. They have taught economic geography, economics and cultural studies at Hunter College CUNY, the University of Southern Maine, and Bates College. They live in Sweden.

About Common Notions

Common Notions is a publishing house and programming platform that fosters new formulations of living autonomy. We aim to circulate timely reflections, clear critiques, and inspiring strategies that amplify movements for social justice.

Our publications trace a constellation of critical and visionary meditations on the organization of freedom. By any media necessary, we seek to nourish the imagination and generalize common notions about the creation of other worlds beyond state and capital. Inspired by various traditions of autonomism and liberation—in the US and internationally, historical and emerging from contemporary movements—our publications provide resources for a collective reading of struggles past, present, and to come.

Common Notions regularly collaborates with political collectives, militant authors, radical presses, and maverick designers around the world. Our political and aesthetic pursuits are dreamed and realized with Antumbra Designs.

www.commonnotions.org
info@commonnotions.org

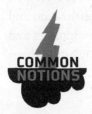